Allergy Products Directory 1995-1996

Asthma Resources Directory

by Carol Rudoff, MA, President, American Allergy Association

Edited by Joann Blessing-Moore, MD
Clinical Assistant Professor, Stanford University Medical Center

Important information. Please read.

This publication is designed to provide general information regarding services and products only. It is violable with the understanding that Allergy Publications, Inc. Is not engaged in rendering any medical or other advice in use or selection. If any medical or other professional assistance is required, the services of a competent physician should be sought.

Throughout this book, trademarked names are used. If a trademark notation was omitted, it was not done to infringe. We use the names only in an editorial fashion, and to the benefit of the trademark owner, with no intention of infringement of the trademark.

Mention of a product or service or facility by name does not constitute or imply an endorsement or recommendation. No product or procedure or location or facility or approach is safe or appropriate for everyone and purchases of products for personal or other use should be discussed with your doctor.

Acceptance of advertisements for publication does not imply endorsement of the products advertised.

This publication and the information contained in these listings was compiled as carefully as possible. Allergy Publications, Inc. cannot guarantee the correctness of all the information contained herein and cannot accept responsibility for omission or errors. The Directory is provided as is.

Offers from previous directories are now replaced by this new publication.

Library of Congress Catalog Card Number: 95-75929
Allergy Products Directory: ISBN 0-944569-02-1
Asthma Resources Directory: ISBN 0-944569-05-6

Acknowledgments

Joann Blessing-Moore, MD

Clinical Assistant Professor

Stanford University Medical Center

Department of Allergy

Private Practice, Allergy and Pediatric Pulmonary

Disease

for reviewing the articles and listings in this directory

Gabriel Groner, PhD

Insight Solutions, Palo Alto, CA

for understanding the complex structure

of this directory and constructing an intelligent

program to create it

Eileen F. Zeller, MPH

Director of Programs, AAFA

Penny Gottier-Fena

Executive Administrator, American Lung Association

"The 'Asthma Resources Directory' is a comprehensive listing of resources and gives many practical tips. It is a gold mine of information for patients and professionals who want to learn more about asthma."

Thomas F. Plaut, MD,
author of *Children with Asthma,*
One Minute Asthma, and the Asthma Diaries.

"Allergy Products Directory" provides easy access to the incredible network of allergy products throughout the United States. This much needed directory has proved to be a tremendous value to the many people that are in search of more information."

Allergy and Asthma Network/
Mothers of Asthmatics, Inc.

Allergy Products Directory

Copyrighted. Reproduction Prohibited by Law. 1259 El Camino #254, Menlo Park, CA 94025

Asthma Resources Directory

Table of Contents

TABLE OF CONTENTS

Asthma Resources Directory

Table of Contents

Asthma Resources Directory

Table of Contents

Allergy Products Directory

Copyrighted. Reproduction Prohibited by Law. 1259 El Camino #254,Menlo Park, CA 94025

Asthma Resources Directory

Table of Contents

Asthma Resources Directory

Table of Contents

Allergy Products Directory

Copyrighted. Reproduction Prohibited by Law. 1259 El Camino #254, Menlo Park, CA 94025

Asthma Resources Directory

How to Use This Directory

HOW TO USE THIS DIRECTORY

INTRODUCTION TO *ALLERGY PRODUCTS DIRECTORY*

Allergy Products Directory lists a wide variety of resources and products that can help individuals and families with their allergy problems.

These resources and products are also of help to the doctors, nurses, respiratory therapists, social workers and dietitians who counsel and treat such individuals and their families.

There are 3897 listings from more than one thousand companies, publishers, and organizations, plus instructive articles, how-to articles, and informative articles that will orient you to the listings.

WHAT'S NEW IN THIS EDITION?

ON LINE ADDRESSES

On-line resources are a new addition to the Directory. You'll find databases, on-line services, discussion groups, bulletin boards, CD-ROM's, and computer programs for the patient and for the professional.

E-MAIL ADDRESSES

Also new is the addition of e-mail addresses when available.

FAX NUMBERS

Fax numbers have been listed when available.

SPANISH LANGUAGE INFORMATION

These publications and education programs have been listed separately for easy referencing.

NUMBER OF CATEGORIES

The number of categories has been greatly increased for more specificity and clarity.

EXPANSION OF ARTICLES

Articles have been re-written, updated, expanded, and corrected in accordance with new medical information, new standards, and new approaches.

Asthma Resources Directory

How to Use This Directory

INCREASE IN NUMBER OF COMPANIES AND LISTINGS

There are many more listings and many more companies listed and these companies and products are cross referenced wherever appropriate.

HOW IS *ALLERGY PRODUCTS DIRECTORY* ARRANGED?

To improve accessibility, the Directory is divided into four Directories, each covering a major topic.

Controlling Your Environment

Here you'll find in-depth articles on assessing and selecting air filters and other products which humidify, dehumidify, heat, and condition your home. Environmental irritants are discussed with suggestions on handling or avoiding them.

The problems with dust and mold in bedroom environments are carefully reviewed with specific suggestions for improvement. Stinging and biting insects are described and steps to take if you are stung are covered in depth along with places to avoid and other precautions. Traveling with allergies has always been difficult. This article discusses how travel affects those with pollen allergy, food allergy, dust and mold allergy, and allergy to environmental smoke.

Listings include filters, dust and pollen controls, mold and mildew aids, specialty stores with mail order catalogues and special services, and titles of books on allergy for adults, children, and professionals.

Allergy/Asthma Finding Help

This volume covers a wide range of help resources with far-ranging capabilities in many areas from organizations to resource centers, telephone information lines, special libraries, newsletters, hospital departments, directories, clearinghouses, emergency preparation and help, patient education programs.

You'll find on line databases, on line services, discussion groups, bulletin boards, CD-ROMs, and computer programs for professionals and for individuals.

Various insurance options are explained and along with standards to evaluate individual and group policies. The

Asthma Resources Directory
How to Use This Directory

SFH's, FFS's, PPO's, HBH's, SFH's and EPO's, are demystified.

Asthma Resources Directory

Today, asthma control involves medication, environmental control, patient education, and measurement of lung function. Medication management evolves during the on-going relationship between you and your doctor. Environmental control is addressed in *Controlling Your Environment.* The last two aspects of management are addressed in this volume.

Asthma triggers, irritant-free pest control, environmental irritants, pulmonary function, and respiratory tools are major explanatory articles. *Talking to Your Doctor* helps you prepare and organize your thoughts and gives you check lists of information your doctor will want to know, and physical signs you should be aware of in order to make decisions about emergency needs, and information the emergency room will need to know.

The article on camps and asthma camps provides you with ideas on evaluating camps and assuring a safe camping experience for your child. You'll also have check lists to assess facilities and programs and information on making your child's experience a productive and meaningful one. The list of specialty camps is arranged by state.

Protecting Your Skin

Offered are two major articles: *Allergic and Irritant Contact Dermatitis* discusses medications, contacts, types of exposures (with special attention to nickel and latex), temperature, foods, even contact lenses solutions and eyeglass frames. Intimate use products and sunscreens are described and *Cosmetics.*

Listings include personal care items (from cosmetics to deodorants) to household products such as cleaning aids and repair products, even shoes and diapers, and specialty stores with mail order catalogues.

Food Allergy Resources (available in 1996)

This volume presents orgaizations, resource centers, hot lines, and health lines that are in-depth

Allergy Products Directory

Copyrighted. Reproduction Prohibited by Law. 1259 El Camino #254, Menlo Park, CA 94025

Asthma Resources Directory

How to Use This Directory

publications and recipe books round out this major source of help.

WHAT KIND OF INFORMATION IS PROVIDED IN A LISTING?

You will find the name of the product, book, program, or resource listed first, an explanation or description, and the companies or publishers or organizations that have that product or resource available. Selection should be made after discussion with your doctor because individual needs and environments vary and should be considered.

The addresses and telephone numbers of companies are supplied with each listing. All cross-referencing is done for you by listing all products, resources, and buying information in each appropriate chapter.

ANTICIPATED AREA CODE CHANGES

In 1995, several area codes changed. Certain sections of area code 206 in Washington state changed to 360; from July 9 you must use the new code. In Alabama certain sections of 205 became 334; from July 16 you must use the new code. In Arizona, Phoenix remained 602 while the rest of the state is 520; from July 23 you must use the new code. In Virginia, area code 703 split to create 540; from July 15 you must use the new code.

HOW DO I FIND WHAT I NEED?

Listings are alphabetized on a word-by-word basis. A listing for *Allergy* will be placed before *AllergyRite.* Companies that use a first name or initial and last name as in *L.L. Bean Co.* are alphabetized on a letter-by-letter basis since this is how the company is known. Names that begin with a number are listed first in order.

Each volume is divided into topic chapters and within those chapters are subheadings of products or services. For example, the section on emergencies is divided into preparing for emergencyes, help during emergencies, emergency communication devices, and travel emergencies.

Under each of those subsections you will find the product name, a description, and the providing company's address, telephone, and fax numbers. Telephone only services will list the service title, a description of the service, and the telephone number.

Asthma Resources Directory
How to Use This Directory

The *Table of Contents* is comprehensive with a list of major headings as well as subheadings. Each chapter begins with its chapter title. Running heads on each page indicate the chapter. The index enables you to go quickly to the specific reference you wish.

POSTAL TWO-LETTER ABBREVIATIONS

We have used the postal service two-letter abbreviations for states, possessions, and Canadian provinces as follows:

Alabama	AL	Ohio	OH
Alaska	AK	Oklahoma	OK
Arizona	AZ	Oregon	OR
Arkansas	AR	Pennsylvania	PA
California	CA	Rhode Island	RI
Colorado	CO	South Carolina	SC
Connecticut	CT	South Dakota	SD
Delaware	DE	Tennessee	TN
Florida	FL	Texas	TX
Georgia	GA	Utah	UT
Hawaii	HI	Vermont	VT
Idaho	ID	Virginia	VA
Illinois	IL	Washington	WA
Indiana	IN	West Virginia	WV
Iowa	IA	Wisconsin	WI
Kansas	KS	Wyoming	WY
Kentucky	KY	District of Columbia	DC
Louisiana	LA	Guam	GU
Maine	ME	Puerto Rico	PR
Maryland	MD	Virgin Islands	VI
Massachusetts	MA		
Michigan	MI		
Minnesota	MN	CANADA	
Mississippi	MS		
Missouri	MO	Alberta	AB
Montana	MT	British Columbia	BC
Nebraska	NE	Manitoba	MB
Nevada	NV	New Brunswick	NB
New Hampshire	NH	Newfoundland	NF
New Jersey	NJ	Nova Scotia	NS
New Mexico	NM	Prince Edward Island	PE
New York	NY	Quebec	PQ
North Carolina	NC	Saskatchewan	SK
North Dakota	ND	NW Territories	NT
		Yukon Territory	YK

Allergy Products Directory
Copyrighted. Reproduction Prohibited by Law. 1259 El Camino #254, Menlo Park, CA 94025

Asthma Resources Directory
Asthma Triggers

ASTHMA TRIGGERS

ALLERGIC AND NON-ALLERGIC TRIGGERS

Triggers are factors or events that have a part in inducing asthma symptoms in people who have asthma or who are susceptible to asthma.

ALLERGENS ARE ALLERGIC TRIGGERS

Allergens are substances that cause allergic reactions when susceptible people come into contact with them by eating (foods), or breathing (pollen, molds), or touching (poison ivies, oaks, cosmetics, metals), or having them injected (drugs).

ENVIRONMENTAL ALLERGENS
OUTDOORS

Outdoors allergens are usually pollen and spores from molds, fungi, mosses and ferns.

POLLEN

Pollen is a predominant cause of outdoor allergic reactions. Allergy-producing pollens come from plants with plain flowers that have a high protein content. Some bee-pollinated plants may also cause problems, although usually their pollen is heavy and not light enough to travel with the winds.

Plain flowers do not attract pollinating bees, so their pollen is light and carried by winds in very high quantities.

Trees usually pollinate in the early to late spring, grasses in the late spring and early summer to fall, and weeds in the late summer and fall until frost. Variations in timing depend on the area and weather patterns.

A pollen count is a measurement of how much pollen there is in an air sample. Sometimes this count can be used to estimate the chances of a person with a specific allergy having an allergy problem where the count was taken. You need to be aware of possible problems with pollen counts.

Asthma Resources Directory

Asthma Triggers

1. Pollen counts are often broadcast after the fact, when the situation may already be different.

2. Pollen may be sampled in one area and then stated for larger areas

3. Pollen counts don't always equal exposure because exposure depends on wind currents, weight of pollens, time of day, rainfall, and how the pollen sample was made.

4. Pollen counts have not been well standardized in the past, but with new programs and training procedures developed by the American Academy of Allergy and Immunology, they may become more useful.

MOLDS

Molds are a cause of seasonal hayfever. Mold proteins, absorbed from molds, travel through the mucous membrane and reach the lungs, causing an allergic asthma attack.

Molds are almost everywhere, outdoors and indoors and can't be avoided. Outdoors, molds live almost anywhere except dry desert regions. They live in fields, forests, at the ocean, on leaf piles, and in compost. Windborne, and numerous after rain, they only disappear after a very hard freeze.

INDOORS

Indoors, allergens are dust mites, cockroaches, pets (dander, saliva, feathers), mold spores, smoke, and plant pollens. If you have problems all year, they are probably caused by indoor allergens.

HOUSE DUST MITES

House dust mites are microscopic arachnids (spider family) that live in huge numbers in your home. (There can be 42,000 mites in one ounce of mattress dust.) House dust mite population increases (by as much as 50%) in the summer as the temperature and humidity levels rise.

There can be 42,000 dust mites in one ounce of mattress dust!

Mites are everywhere, including beaches and mountain areas. In areas where it is very dry, there are fewer dust mites. Even when mite populations are low, you can suffer symptoms because their dried body parts and their fecal matter remain.

Asthma Resources Directory

Asthma Triggers

Dust mites are closely associated with human skin scales, so we cannot escape them. They are an integral part of house dust, blending with spores, animal skin flakes, disintegrated stuffing materials from pillows, mattresses, blankets, draperies, upholstered furniture, and carpets, even toys.

COCKROACHES

Cockroaches are strong allergens. The specific source of an allergen is the dried parts of the cockroach body. Asthmatic individuals with many allergies can develop cockroach sensitivity.

PETS

Pet dander or skin flakes are an allergic component of house dust, they are also an allergen by themselves. Dander is a long-lasting problem. It can remain in a home on furniture, carpets, and floors that has not had a pet for months, even years.

Your pet's dander or skin flakes, saliva, and urine are allergens and also an allergic part of house dust.

Animal saliva, especially from cats, is another problem. Cats clean themselves, covering their fur with saliva. These very small saliva proteins (Fel d1) can remain airborne for hours, enter the lungs and causing asthma symptoms.If your dog licks you, its protein saliva will transfer to your skin. If you are very sensitive, your skin may turn red and itch where your pet licks you.

Cat allergen also comes from glands that produce oil and there are dog allergens in urine and saliva as well as dander.

MOLDS

Molds are a part of our home environment. Mold growth is almost everywhere in homes where it is damp. Molds grow wherever there is moisture: in bathrooms, on foods, on furniture, plants, wallpaper, refrigerator gaskets, basements, humidifiers, air conditioners, and attics.

Asthma Resources Directory
Asthma Triggers

FOODS AND ADDITIVES

Food allergy is a hypersensitivity to specific foods. Eating these foods causes local symptoms like an upset stomach, a stuffy nose or systemic symptoms like a rash and even wheezing or life-threatening reactions.

Additives, including MSG, sulfites, and colorings can be troublesome to some people, and have been reported to cause bronchospasm or anaphylaxis in those with severe asthma.

Foods with mold can include, but are not limited to, beer, wine, yeast-baked products, buttermilk, sour cream, non-processed cheeses, cider, dried fruits, mushrooms, sauerkraut, smoked meats and fish, hot dogs, sausages, corned beef, vinegar and foods with vinegar.

Additives like MSG, sulfites, and food colorings can be troublesome

Foods with sulfites can include, but are not limited to, lemon juice, dried fruits, wine, molasses, grape juice, wine vinegar, instant potatoes, and fresh shrimp. Some of these foods like dried fruits, fresh shrimp, and lemon juice may contain sulfites.

As of August, 1987, Food and Drug Administration (FDA) banned use of sulfite preservatives in fresh vegetables and fruits sold in food stores and restaurants. This ban did not apply to prepared potatoes that are sold to restaurants or to consumers in supermarkets, nor to dried fruit, shrimp, or wine.

In 1990, sulfite use was banned on produce and fruits in salad bars. In storage, potatoes in skins can be sprayed with sulfites. Unfortunately, FDA lost a court case, so fries and hash browns can be made with potatoes treated with sulfites after peeling.

NON-ALLERGIC ASTHMA TRIGGERS
IRRITANTS

Irritants are potentially a problem for anyone, but when your airways are hypersensitive, you're more likely to react.

FUMES AND ODORS

Inhaled substances can seriously affect health. They can trigger symptoms even though they are not allergens.

9

Asthma Resources Directory

Asthma Triggers

Strong fumes are particularly likely to cause nasal symptoms because they irritate the mucous membranes of the nose. Some fumes can make your allergic rhinitis or asthma worse. If you have asthma, try to avoid tobacco smoke and substances that are easily vaporized.

AIR AT HOME

Air at home can affect your asthma. Fumes from cooking odors like fish can cause problems as well as indoor combustion from gas fireplaces and stoves. Mothballs and flakes, floor wax, and cleaners, liquid chlorine bleach, furniture polish, room deodorizers, deodorants, perfumes, hair sprays, talcum powders, scented cosmetics, aerosols, and tobacco smoke are other sources of irritating odors at home.

The odor of a new vinyl mattress cover can give you a headache or watery eyes. Christmas trees can cause an asthmatic reaction in some very sensitive individuals. Some resinous woods are irritating and when burned in your fireplace can cause eye irritation. There is also the risk of coughing from released particulates.

AIR AT WORK

Air we breathe while at work may be an important cause of asthma for many people. Try to avoid strong chemical and paint fumes, and, gasoline, diesel, and kerosene fumes, insecticide sprays, newly printed newspapers, wax, cleaning fluid, with chlorine and ammonia, brass polishers, tobacco smoke, printing ink, cleaning solvents, paints, glues, paint thinner, and sprays, cleaners.

The air we breathe while at work may be an important cause of asthma for many.

Occupational Dusts and Vapors from working with plastics, grains, fertilizers, metals, and woods can be a problem. Sometimes masks and respirators help, but sometimes retraining or transfer must be considered.

If you experience chest discomfort while you are working, you should be concerned. Don't ignore this discomfort as job-related tension. It could be the beginning of an airway obstruction. If you have a peak flow meter, use it before and after exposure and consult with your doctor.

POLLUTANTS

Pollutants can remain in the air for days or even weeks, especially in cities. Some pollutants increase airway

Allergy Products Directory
Copyrighted. Reproduction Prohibited by Law. 1259 El Camino #254, Menlo Park, CA 94025

Asthma Resources Directory
Asthma Triggers

reactivity even in normal people and pollutants can irritate the airways. Examples of some common irritants that are especially troublesome for people with asthma are cigarette smoke, newsprint, and cold air.

While in a car, be aware that fumes in heavy traffic, particularly if cars do not have smog control devices can be very irritating. Driving in tunnels and in cities with high density buildings, or being stuck in a traffic jam can bring on symptoms because of poor quality air.

WHAT TO DO WHEN DRIVING

- Avoid travel during rush hour

- If you must drive under adverse conditions, keep your windows closed, especially during pollen season

- Use an air conditioner that recirculates inner air

- Covering the car air vents with cheese cloth (and change it frequently) while operating the air conditioner may help minimize symptoms that you may suffer from because of mold growth in the air conditioning system

- Vacuum the car frequently, using a protective mask

- Keep doors and windows closed at gasoline stations and use a protective mask

- In states with self-service gas pumps, pay to have the attendant fill your tank

WHAT TO DO ABOUT POLLUTANTS IN THE AIR

Pollutants in the air like ozone, carbon monoxide, sulfur dioxide, and nitrogen dioxide are damaging to be exposed to and more damaging if you are exercising or working.

- Keep current on air quality (radio, TV, newspaper)

- Exercise early when pollutant levels (including pollens) are lower

- Do not exercise when air pollution levels are high

- Don't exercise near heavily used roads, especially if there is stalled traffic

- If symptoms occur, stop exercising immediately

HELP US TO HELP YOU

When writing to the companies and organizations listed here, be sure to use the initials (APD) as part of the address and tell them you saw them listed in *Allergy Products Directory.*

11

Asthma Resources Directory

Asthma Triggers

COLD AIR CONDITIONS

Cold, dry air causes problems for many with asthma. Your airways become dry and cooler. This may contribute to wheezing during the rewarming. Try to protect your mouth and nose by keeping them warm with mufflers or head gear. There are several products which may be of help.

COLD AIR PROTECTION

AirClear Mask® is made of polyfoam. It covers the nose, not the head and comes in adult and children's sizes. It is available from: *The Pulmonary Paper* at 800-950-3698.

Airgard™ is handwashable and can fit below glasses frames. It is available from Airgard, Inc. At 219-457-5237

Blo-Go Heat Exchanger uses a different approach. It has a mouthpiece connected to a respiratory heat and humidity exchanger; on initial respiration, exchanger is cooled; during exhalation, exchanger is warmed and water vapor condenses on it; on the next inhalation, cold air passes over the warm, moist exchanger and is warmed and humidified; the exchanger is cooled and dried, ready to trap the heat and moisture of the next exhalation. It is available from Vacumetrics, Vacu-Med at 800-235-3333.

Spenco® Cold Air Mask has a breathing chamber that warms inhaled air to a minimum of 60°F and increases relative humidity to 95%. It is available from Allergy Asthma Technology 800-621-5545.

WEATHER CONDITIONS

There is a great deal of pollen in the air during windy weather and you may find that your symptoms increase during this time. If there is little wind along with temperature inversions, smog is trapped and pollution indices are high.

Rain reduces the amount of allergens, irritants, and pollutants in the air, but rain means more mold spores. Summer rains can result in higher ragweed pollen production in late summer and early fall.

When the weather is dry, pollens remain airborne longer. In hot weather, grasses produce more pollens.

12

Asthma Resources Directory

Asthma Triggers

INFECTIONS

Viral infections or colds and the flu can develop into a wheeze or cough for an asthmatic person because the viral infection makes the airways more sensitive. Viruses, by damaging the lining of the airways, stimulate sensory nerve fibers. They also increase permeability of the airway mucous membrane for other irritants and allergens triggering asthma.

Viral infections are an important cause of wheezing in individuals with sensitive lungs. After a viral infection, the airways may remain more reactive to viruses and irritants.

Breathing rapidly, as when emotionally upset, can allow enough cold dry air to pass over the moist mucous membranes to cool and irritate them, producing asthma symptoms.

EXERCISE-INDUCED BRONCHOSPASM

Exercise can cause wheezing. This is known as exercise-induced bronchospasm.

Most people with allergic asthma will wheeze during or following exercise. They may experience wheezing, coughing, and chest tightness five to ten minutes after exercise or later. The wheezing will be worse from two to five minutes and then decrease in intensity with or without treatment.

Viral infection makes the airways more sensitive.

Viral infections are an important cause of wheezing in individuals with sensitive lungs.

Exercising and breathing with your mouth open allows cool, dry air to pass over the moist mucous membranes, causing the membranes to lose moisture and creating heat loss. This cools the airways, irritating them, and on rewarming, an asthmatic attack occurs. Even breathing rapidly, as when emotionally upset, can allow enough cold dry air to pass over the moist mucous membranes and produce symptoms.

Exercising with your mouth open allows cool, dry air to pass over the moist mucous membranes in your lungs.

The membranes lose moisture and cool, become irritated, and on rewarming, an asthmatic attack occurs

13

Asthma Resources Directory

Asthma Triggers

Environmental contributors to wheezing after exercise are smog, pollen, and cold weather. Take medication before exercising, do a complete warm-up, and don't exercise when environmental contributors are present.

ANAPHYLAXIS

Anaphylaxis is a severe, life-threatening allergic reaction requiring immediate medical attention.

A reaction may start out as mild or severe. The sooner the symptoms occur, the more severe the reaction. Early feelings include uneasiness, weakness, itching, sneezing, sweating, and hives. These are followed by difficulty in breathing, wheezing, difficulty in swallowing (because of swelling of tissues), vomiting, stomach pain, fainting, or shock. More severe reactions may be a need to urinate or incontinence, loss of bowel control, convulsions, coma. Bronchospasms can close off breath and death may follow.

EXERCISE-INDUCED ANAPHYLAXIS

The severity of the wheezing seems to be related to how strenuous the activity is. In many patients, the symptoms are very mild, a cough or tight feeling in the chest. In other patients, wheezing is severe enough to require treatment.

Exercise training does raise the threshold for exertion before significant wheezing is noted.

According to Dr. Joann Blessing-Moore, training does not seem to lessen the attacks for the asthmatic child. However, exercise training does raise the threshold for exertion before significant wheezing is noted. It is important for families and teachers to be aware of the potential wheezing, coughing or chest tightness that can occur with strenuous exercise.

FOOD-DEPENDENT, EXERCISE-INDUCED ANAPHYLAXIS

Food-dependent, exercise-induced anaphylaxis is rare. Some individuals may suffer anaphylaxis when they exercise after eating. Some may experience an anaphylactic reaction only if they have eaten certain foods and then exercised.

Faye Dong, RD, PhD reported on two cases where eating celery and then exercising caused anaphylaxis and a third

Allergy Products Directory
Copyrighted. Reproduction Prohibited by Law. 1259 El Camino #254,Menlo Park, CA 94025

Asthma Resources Directory
Asthma Triggers

case where the patient exercised and later ate celery resulting in anaphylaxis.

If reaction to celery is severe, it should be completely eliminated from the diet. When eating out, avoid salads with celery and sandwiches like chicken salad and egg salad. Check with the kitchen to be sure your food does not contain celery. If you have *any* doubt, do not eat the dish.

Dr. Thomas M. Golbert has written about individuals who experience exercise-induced anaphpylaxis *only* when they exercised within two hours of eating.

Dr. Goldbert notes that one group develops anaphylaxis no matter what they have eaten and the other group can tie their anaphylaxis to a particular food.

Doctors recommend:

✔ Dont exercise for at least three hours after you eat

✔ Talk to your doctor about carrying epinephrine

✔ Exercise with a friend

MISCELLANEOUS

Miscellaneous items causing asthma include cottonseed, kapok, flaxseed for stuffing pillows, furniture, sleeping bags, and stuffed animals.

ASPIRIN, SULFITES AND DYES

Aspirin: The mechanism is not understood, but some asthma sufferers are intolerant to aspirin. Some asthma patients who have used aspirin notice that breathing becomes more difficult after taking it. It is therefore recommended that people with asthma avoid aspirin. Read medication labels carefully because aspirin is present in many products, including most over-the-counter preparations pain remedies.

Drugs like acetaminophen (Tylenol) are rarely a cause of asthma. Check with your doctor before using.

People with asthma should avoid nonsteroidal anti-inflammatory drugs to reduce pain and inflammation. They can cause the same asthmatic symptoms as aspirin. These medications include drugs sold under the brand names:

Asthma Resources Directory

Asthma Triggers

Advil
Anaprox
butazolidin
Clinoril
Feldene
Indocin
Meclomen
Motrin
Nalfron
Naposyn
Nuprin
rufen
Tolectin

Drugs like acetaminophen (Tylenol) are rarely a cause of asthma, so if you are aspirin sensitive, you may be able to use acetaminophen products safely. And as with any medication decision, ask your doctor if you are uncertain.

Sulfites: FDA banned the use of sulfites on fresh fruits and vegetables in restaurants and markets in 1986. Sulfites are usually not used on meat products or fish, other than shellfish. Also implicated are potassium or sodium bisulfite, potassium or sodium metabisulfite, sodium sulfite, and sulfur dioxide.

As of 1987, warning statements are included in the labeling of all prescription drugs which have sulfites added to the final dosage, even as an inactive ingredient. Sulfites are not completely prohibited because they maintain the potency of certain medications, some of which can save lives.

As of 1987, warning statements are included in the labeling of all prescription drugs which have sulfites added to the final dosage as an inactive ingredient.

Sulfites are used in extremely small amounts in manufacturing hard gelatin capsules. Sulfite reactions to these capsules are very uncommon. This means that many drug products that have not had sulfites added as inactive ingredients may contain some level of sulfite from indirect sources. The FDA rule does not apply to such products. It applies only to prescription products to which sulfites have been directly added as an inactive ingredient.

Asthma Resources Directory

Asthma Triggers

> **Drinking wine can trigger asthma symptoms from sulfites in wine that inhibit bacterial growth. Even if winemakers do not add sulfites, they are produced naturally by the action of yeast during fermentation.**

Dyes: Antihistamines that are liquids and pills may be colored by dyes, which can cause allergic reactions. Capsules generally have fewer additives. In addition to the pure FD&C dyes, various combinations may be used to blend other colors. Ask your doctor or pharmacist, or ask the manufacturer which dyes have been used.

White antihistamines may be free of all dyes. Check before using as formulas may change.

HELP US TO HELP YOU

When writing to the companies and organizations listed here, be sure to use the initials (APD) as part of the address and tell them you saw them listed in *Allergy Products Directory.*

If you call, be sure to tell them you found them in *Allergy Products Directory.*

Thank you for your help.

17

Asthma Resources Directory

Home Environment

YOUR HOME ENVIRONMENT

Perennial rhinitis and asthma are very common respiratory complaints. Rhinitis symptoms include runny and stuffy nose, itching eyes, sore throat, sneezing, coughing, and, perhaps, sinusitis. Asthma symptoms include wheezing, coughing, difficulty breathing (especially at night), and difficulty breathing from exercise, strong odors, or cold air or allergic causes.

Controlling the indoor environment is very important since we spend the vast majority of our time indoors and a very large part of that indoor time in our bedrooms.

Sometimes eczema, a skin allergy that results in a rash that itches and is red, develops from exposure to preservatives in products, oils, and resins, or plant products.

Controlling the indoor environment is very important since we spend the vast majority of our time indoors (at home, shopping, at recreational and entertainment events, or at work) and a very large part of that indoor time in our bedrooms.

HOUSE DUST MITES

House dust is a mixture of house dust mite protein, the dander from your pets, cockroaches, molds, outdoor pollen, and spores. Dust mites (*Dermatophagoides pteronyssinus*) are so small they can only be seen through a microscope. They are arachnids (in the same family as spiders) and live in mattresses, bedding, carpets, upholstery, clothing, and anything with fabric, especially nubby and textured fabrics, even stuffed toys.

One female dust mite can lay up to 50 eggs every three weeks!

Dusts fall on and cling to heavily upholstered and overstuffed furniture and flocked wallpapers. They live on human skin scales and so live anywhere that we live.

It is the waste products and body parts of the mites to which most people react. Since one female mite can lay up to 50 eggs every three weeks, your bed alone can be host to untold numbers. These are persistent and numerous adversaries.

Asthma Resources Directory

Home Environment

Avoid carpeting where possible. Vacuuming stirs up and scatters dust. Mites have sticky pads on their feet that cling strongly to surfaces, so vacuuming is generally not effective at removing live mites, but does remove the feces and body parts that can be inhaled. When you walk on the carpet, mite waste matter floats up and can be inhaled and cause allergic symptoms. Therefore, you should vacuum thoroughly and often even though you are not getting rid of the mites themselves, you are removing mite feces and body parts.

Mites have sticky pads on their feet that cling strongly to surfaces, so vacuuming is generally not effective at removing live mites, but does remove the feces and body parts that can be inhaled.

When you make the bed or air it out or change sheets, you are disturbing mite waste matter and may experience symptoms. Washing in hot water is effective in keeping mite populations down.

You will want to strive for a clean, uncluttered look. Only keep display items that you really love. Don't try to fill every square inch of space. Consider displaying in glass-door cabinets. Hardwood and tile flooring have a beautiful look and can be damp mopped. Make it easy for yourself to keep your rooms clean.

PREPARING AND MAINTAINING THE BEDROOM

If you have a family history of this type of allergy problem, it is a good idea to prepare and maintain the bedroom before your child is born. It is still a good idea even if a child has no symptoms. According to Dr. Joann Blessing-Moore, there are good data to indicate that such precautions can delay the onset of allergies.

You will want to concentrate on keeping your bedroom or the bedrooms of your allergic children as dust free as you can because so many hours are spent in the bedroom. This can be done by isolating the bedroom as much as possible from the air circulation pattern of the house. Keep the doors and windows closed at all times. Install a window air conditioner if you don't have central air conditioning. Keep pets out. Remember, most doctors prefer you find your pet another home.

Asthma Resources Directory

Home Environment

Do not pull up carpeting with your allergic child home.

Reactions can be severe.

With care and planning, you may find that symptoms can diminish considerably in this room and that it can be used during the day for other activities as well as for moments of relief.

If you or your child have severe problems, adapt the Japanese way of leaving your shoes outside the bedroom so as not to track in outdoor grime.

If at all possible, empty the bedroom and remove the carpeting. **Do not pull up and remove the carpeting with your allergic child at home. Reactions can be severe.** If you have hardwood floors, just clean them and enjoy their beauty. Otherwise, if you can, select vinyl or linoleum. They are easier to keep clean and will not harbor dust mites.

Everything that goes into a bedroom should be needed and easily washable, including, rugs, drapes, bedspread, blankets, or comforters.

Clean the walls, the floor, and ceiling; the windows, window sills, and molding; the closet, the light fixtures, and door molding. Clean the radiator. You can cover forced hot-air heating vents with a double layer of cheesecloth to trap larger particles, but cheesecloth will not trap pollen. Cheesecloth should be replaced at least weekly. More often is better. You may also use replaceable fiber glass or plastic filters. Replace them monthly.

Everything that goes into a bedroom should be needed and should be easily washable, including, rugs, drapes, bedspread, blankets, or comforters. The bedroom should be completely cleaned once a week, including mopping the floor and cleaning the walls and window sills.

Toys should be washable and preferably made of wood, plastic, or metal; if favorite stuffed toys remain, they must be hot water washable and dryable in the drier. Keep them in the dryer for at least 45 minutes. Store stuffed toys each night, preferably in a plastic bag. Do not leave them on a shelf.

The bedroom should be completely cleaned once a week, including mopping the floor and cleaning the walls and window sills.

The good news here is that Abstract #440 at the American Academy of Allergy meeting, March 12-17, 1993

Asthma Resources Directory

Home Environment

indicated that velour blanket squares put into a dryer for at least 45 minutes was effective in lowering mite population from an average of 547 mites in an 8-inch square to 8 mites in an 8-inch square. This means that a favorite stuffed toy or blankets which cannot take extensive washings *may* be effectively treated in the dryer only. Talk to your doctor.

The following article is an in-depth look at what you can do to make your child's bedroom or your own bedroom as comfortable and as allergen-free as possible. Specific aspects of the bedroom environment are explored with specific action suggestions. (Products mentioned are found in our listings.)

RUG

As it is the largest potential collector of dust in the bedroom, make every effort to remove the carpet and its underlying pad which can also support mold. **Remember: Do not pull up the carpeting with your allergic child at home. Reactions can be severe.**

When installing new carpeting in other areas of the house, use a low-emitting adhesive if adhesives are needed. Try to be outside during installation and stay away for a while after installation. Open doors and windows during installation. If you have fans or an air conditioner, use them for a couple of days after installation.

Vacuuming does not lower your live dust mite population because live mites cling to the carpet fibers.

Vacuuming does not lower your live dust mite population. Live mites cling to the carpet fibers. Vacuuming will decrease mite feces and body parts which can be stirred up and inhaled when walking.

✔ Vacuum while your allergic child is at school

✔ If you are allergic to dust and must do the vacuuming, be sure to wear a mask with an appropriate level of protection while you vacuum

✔ Don't take your mask off as soon as you finish because your vacuuming will have stirred up all sorts of problem-causing particles that can float around for at least 15 minutes

✔ Investigate a central vacuum system that is vented outdoors or investigate a vacuum with high efficiency filters.

Asthma Resources Directory

Home Environment

✔ Another possible solution is to use disposable plastic drop cloths found at paint stores. Tape them over your old rug. If you leave your shoes outside the door, your plastic rug may last a week or two.

✔ A spray that keep the dust mite population down are also available

FLOOR

When you remove old carpeting in an older home, you may discover hardwood floors beneath. These are easier to keep clean than carpets.

> **WARNING—** Do not pull up the carpeting with your allergic child or anyone with a severe reaction in the house. The reaction can be serious. Stay away from the house for as long as possible.

If you have tile, it is not only attractive, it makes a good playing floor and spills from crafts projects, snacks, and accidents wipe up easily. If you use a throw rug, it should be lintless cotton that you can easily wash each week. If your floor is in poor condition, cover it with linoleum or vinyl and use molding to seal spaces between the baseboard and the floor. Mop weekly and twice a month, damp mop with a disinfectant solution that fights mold. One part chlorine bleach to 10 parts water is a good disinfectant.

BED

Since we spend the most hours in bed, do not place your bed in line with the air vent because dust and molds can be blown into the room through the vent by the heating and cooling systems.

Avoid bunk beds.

The upper bed is more difficult to clean and dust can fall on the lower bed.

Avoid bunk beds. The upper bed is more difficult to clean and dust can fall on the lower bed. If you must use bunk beds, remember to cover the mattresses and pillows on both beds and do not keep stuffed animals on the upper bunk. Do not use the upper bunk for storage of any kind.

Your mattress should be synthetic. The bed should be of metal or wood. First, thoroughly clean the bed frame and springs. Try to vacuum the bed frame at least monthly,

Allergy Products Directory
Copyrighted. Reproduction Prohibited by Law. 1259 El Camino #254, Menlo Park, CA 94025

Asthma Resources Directory
Home Environment

preferably, more often. Thoroughly vacuum and dust the bedsprings.

MATTRESS ENCASINGS

Since dust mites flourish in your mattress, a cover or case made of plastic or vinyl (not cotton) with a zipper should enclose it. Cover the full length of the zipper with wide masking tape. You can use a washable, cotton mattress pad under the sheet. Be sure to also cover the box spring.

PILLOWS

Your pillows should be a non-allergenic, washable synthetic like dacron or polyester. Look for a "hypoallergenic" label and wash your pillow weekly in hot water and dry in a hot dryer. Encase it inside a plastic or vinyl cover and cover the zipper with wide masking tape.

Feather pillows can't be washed and are allergens in their own right. They also contain dust mites and mold. Even if you encase a feather pillow, the dust-proof cover will only protect you from dust mites, not from feather allergens.

Even if you encase a feather pillow, the dust-proof cover will only protect you from dust mites not from feather allergens.

If you use foam rubber pillows, they must be replaced every few months or at least annually because they disintegrate and because molds can grow on them.

SHEETS AND PILLOWCASES

Cotton is preferred. When you change the sheets, vacuum the encasings that are on the pillows, mattress, and box springs and sponge them clean.

BLANKETS AND BEDSPREADS

Blankets should be synthetic or cotton and washed weekly. Avoid woolen blankets and down comforters. The bedspread should also be cotton or a washable synthetic, and both should have a smooth finish. Be sure to wash with hot water and dry bedding in a dryer if available. Heat kills mites.

Asthma Resources Directory

Home Environment

CEILING AND WALLS

If possible, the walls and ceiling should be smooth, without a finish and without a wallpaper that collects dust. After washing thoroughly with a mild water and bleach combination of one part chlorine bleach to 10 parts water, ceilings and walls may be painted or papered with a washable wallpaper. Be sure to use mildew-resistant adhesive. Vacuum the ceiling and walls monthly.

WINDOWS AND WINDOW TREATMENT

In humid climtes, and when pollen and mold are problems, keep the windows closed. The windows should fit tightly. Use weather stripping. Install a window air conditioner if you don't have central air conditioning.

Sheets make colorful, washable, and easily replaceable curtains.

Venetian blinds and shutters collect dust and are not easily cleaned. Bright, colorful curtains that can easily be taken down weekly and laundered are best. Sheets make colorful, washable curtains. They work well and can be colorful accessories in a child's room and sophisticated color accents in an adult room

Window shades provide privacy and light control. They can be laminated with fabrics that match bedspreads and are available in contrasting or harmonizing colors. Shades will need to be wiped with a mild disinfectant solution that prevents mold. Be sure to wipe both sides of the shade. If you live in a high humidity area, you may find you need to use this mold preventive weekly.

FURNITURE

Furniture should have simple lines and not be ornate with grooves that catch dust. A desk chair should be a washable vinyl or plastic. Heavily upholstered furniture

---

Avoid ornate furniture with grooves that catch dust.

---

and pillows can be champion collectors of dust and don't belong in the bedroom. Padding should be a foam plastic. Remember that kapok and feathers can produce allergens and foam rubber supports mold. Twice a month wipe the vinyl with a disinfectant solution that fights mold like one part chlorine bleach to 10 parts water.

Allergy Products Directory
Copyrighted. Reproduction Prohibited by Law. 1259 El Camino #254, Menlo Park, CA 94025

Asthma Resources Directory
Home Environment

BOOKS

Books and bibelots are dust collectors and support mold growth. Either store them in another room or put them, and any magazines, inside a cabinet with doors.

PICTURES

If you are willing to clean and dust them each week, you can hang pictures. Pennants can contain hair and should taken down from bedrooms walls.

DOOR

Try to keep the bedroom door closed all the time.

CLOSETS

Closets are a part of the room. Think of the bedroom closet as a room in your bedroom and treat it exactly as you do the bedroom. Bedroom closets are also dust collectors that can spew dust into the bedroom air whenever you fling open the door.

Don't store anything in the closet.

Keep only clothes currently in use.

Don't store items in the closet, especially books. Keep only clothes currently in use in the closet. If you must store clothing in the closet, store it in plastic bags without mothballs or camphor. Keep shoes on a shoe rack that you can easily remove from the closet so that you can clean the floors and corners. When you clean the bedroom, clean the closet, the closet floor, and then close its door.

AIR CLEANER

These are discussed elsewhere in *Allergy Products Directory*. Air cleaners cannot take the place of environmental controls in your home and if you use them, they should be used along with the methods discussed above and not instead of.

HUMIDITY

Dust mites do not survive at humidity levels less than 20%. The more humid the air in your home is, the more

Asthma Resources Directory

Home Environment

dust mites you will have, so try to keep the humidity level in your home low. Thirty-five to 45% humidity may be a good compromise, although some sources prefer lower. As a rule of thumb, if the outdoor temperature is 40°, inside humidity should be 45%; if outdoor temperature is 0 degrees, inside humidity should be 25%.

Keeping the room temperature below 70°
and room humidity below 50% helps to control dust mites.

Keeping the room temperature below 70° and room humidity below 50% helps to control dust mites. During showering or cooking, use an exhaust fan.

Air conditioners can help keep your mite population down by removing excess humidity from the atmosphere. An electric blanket or sheet on 'low' during the day keeps the dust mite population in your bed low also.

PETS

Pets should not be allowed in the bedroom and should be kept out of the house. Many doctors prefer that their patients not keep pets at all. It takes many, many months for dander to dissipate from your home.

HEATING/COOLING SYSTEMS AND DUCTWORK

Try to make the bedroom independent of the household's heating and cooling systems. You can then use separate heating units, air conditioners, and air filters to control dust and mold and keep the room much cleaner with less effort.

If you have a forced air heating system, use a special dust filter on the furnace and install an air purifier. Furnaces and cooling systems trap dust and dirt. In order for them to function efficiently, their filters must either be cleaned or changed frequently. Filters and purifiers are discussed elsewhere in *Allergy Products Directory*.

If you have a forced air heating system,
use a special dust filter on the furnace and install an air purifier.

Furnaces and cooling systems trap dust and dirt.

In the fall, before starting your heating system, clean or vacuum the registers thoroughly. In the summer, before

Asthma Resources Directory

Home Environment

starting your cooling system, clean or vacuum the registers thoroughly; otherwise, months of accumulated dust and molds can be spewed into your home.

Electric heat is the cleanest. Avoid fans and blowers in favor of radiation or convection heating units.

Keep your air conditioner and dehumidifier scrupulously clean and free of mold

Air conditioners and dehumidifiers seem to help keep mite population low by removing excess water (humidity) from the atmosphere. These units must be kept scrupulously clean and free of mold and bacteria growth. (See *Living with the Air in Your Home* in this Directory.)

LIVING AREAS

In theory, you would like to handle other main living areas as though they were bedrooms. Remove moldy carpet pads and carpets, take down draperies, remove stuffed furniture and pillows, pack away accessories, and keep only those special items that you are willing to keep scrupulously clean.

As a practical matter, cast a careful eye over your living areas. If you have a family room, you probably spend a fair amount of time there and so do your children. It may be the kind of room you would tackle next. If the carpeting is old, consider replacing it with tile that can handle spills and scuffing when your children play. Tile is also easily mopped.

Tackle your family room next.

You and your family spend a great deal of time in it.

For other living areas (dining room or dining area, living room, den, sunroom) consider how you can replace aging carpets, drapes, stuffed furniture, pillows. Save your budget for replacing major items like carpeting. Can you use area rugs? Is there a wood floor under the old carpet? Is there a tile flooring that will give your home a new look?

MOLD CONTROL - INDOOR MOLDS

Mildew is a fungus that grows as a surface mold on just about anything. Mildew spores are in the air waiting for a welcoming environment: warm and moist.

Allergy Products Directory

Copyrighted. Reproduction Prohibited by Law. 1259 El Camino #254, Menlo Park, CA 94025

Asthma Resources Directory

Home Environment

Where there are warmth, moisture (humidity) and darkness, there are molds. You can smell them. They have a musty odor which experience has taught us to associate with mildew. You can sometimes see where mildew has discolored a material.

Wherever you find warmth, moisture, and darkness, you'll find mold.

To eliminate molds, you must eliminate the conditions that encourage them. Ventilating rooms and closets and lighting them keeps them dry and inhibits mold formation. Lowering the humidity level to below 40 percent contributes to an environment that does not encourage mold.

MILDEW ON WALLS

If your walls are mildewed, don't paint over them. The mildew will grow through the new paint. Instead, wash the wall. Try one of the following:

One ounce of bleach in three quarts of water. Let the mixture dry on the wall surface for 20 minutes, then rinse thoroughly with fresh water. Let the wall dry before painting.

Add one quart liquid chlorine bleach to three quarts of warm water. Stir in one-third cup powdered laundry detergent. Apply with a sponge or nylon brush. Leave on long enough for the black stains to turn white, but don't let it dry. Rinse thoroughly and then let dry. (U.S. Dept. of Agriculture)

> **WARNING — Do not mix bleach with ammonia. The combination can release a poisonous gas**

Ask at the paint store about paint additives that may help control mildewing. Some exterior paints may be formulated with such additives in them.

BASEMENT

To control dampness in basements, use an electric heater or dehumidifier or, if possible, leave screened windows opened. Keep an incandescent light burning. Humidity levels should be maintained between 30 and 50%. Repair and water proof concrete or cinder block walls.

Ask a building contractor about plastic shields under cement flooring and for closet walls. Do not use a basement

Asthma Resources Directory

Home Environment

as a living area unless it does not leak, is dry and mold-free and has sufficient ventillation. Avoid carpets. They can become moldy rapidly.

BATHROOMS

In your bathrooms, window sills, shower stalls, shower curtains, and tile grout encourage mold growth. Scrub this growth with a brush dipped in a liquid bleach solution or commercially available mold-preventive. (See *Fighting Mold.*) Use paint in your bathroom rather than wallpaper and give mold less of a hiding place.

Use paint in your bathroom rather than wallpaper and give mold less of a hiding place.

Replace shower curtains that are mildewed. Carpeting in the bathroom develops mold rapidly and should be avoided. If the room doesn't have a vent fan, install one or keep the window opened. After the family's bathing and showering is done, leave the bathroom door opened and the vent fan going until the humidity level is down.

CLOSETS

Damp closets can be helped by installing fans, louvered doors, opening windows, burning an incandescent light, or using a small dehumidifier.

KITCHEN

Cooking raises the level of moisture in the air, supporting mold growth, while use of cleaning chemicals, storage of cleaning chemicals and leftover products, placement of household plants (See below.), and pest

---

Cooking raises the level of moisture in the air, supporting mold growth.

Use the exhaust fan when cooking and cleaning.

---

control procedures mean following careful steps to keep the kitchen clear of indoor pollutants. Use the exhaust fan when cooking and cleaning. Do not use the oven to heat the room. Discard old or unused chemical products. Read the chapter on non-irritating pest control.

Allergy Products Directory

Copyrighted. Reproduction Prohibited by Law. 1259 El Camino #254, Menlo Park, CA 94025

Asthma Resources Directory

Home Environment

If your laundry equipment is in the area, be sure the clothes dryer vents outdoors. Turn on ventilating fans while using laundry equipment.

REFRIGERATOR

Molds or mildew grow on the gasket around the inside of the refrigerator door. Inside the refrigerator, you'll find mold on spoiled fruit or old cheese. Keep refrigerators clean and

throw out spoiled food. Do not try to cut away mold that you can see and save the rest of the food. The mold has penetrated rest of the food and none of it should be eaten.

More recent thought is that larger foods with the mold cut away leaving a broad, clean border may be safe to eat. Smaller foods like grapes should be thrown away if mold is on them. Consider the cost and replaceability of the item and err on the side of caution.

Protect yourself by wearing a mask with an appropriate level of protection or have someone else clean the dusty coils of the refrigerator. You'll save money on the cost of running the appliance.

TRASH COMPACTOR

Don't neglect regular cleaning of your trash compactor. It will encourage mold, especially in warmer weather, when you may notice a distinctly unpleasant odor. Let the container air in full sunlight or wash thoroughly with soap and let dry completely.

PLANTS

Molds also grow on the surface of clay pots, dead leaves, and on the soil of your house plants. Depending upon your degree of sensitivity, you may need to scrub the clay pots, keep your plants free of dead leaves, and put charcoal on the soil, or you may try growing cactus, or you may have to give your plants away. Also consider that any water spillage on carpeting and padding will support mold growth.

ATTIC MILDEW

Attics need ventilation (roof fan or louvers) as well as a vapor barrier. Activities like showering, bathing, cooking, or laundering, produce a great deal of moisture that is absorbed into the air of your home. Your home needs sufficient ventilation for water vapor to escape.

Asthma Resources Directory

Home Environment

Your home needs sufficient ventilation for water vapor to escape.

Older homes, probably built without vapor barriers, are vulnerable to moisture in the air, and condensation.

Unfortunately, the newer homes of today are more energy-efficient and tightly sealed. There are usually not as many air exchanges per hour as older, more leaky houses are likely to have. When windows must be kept closed because of pollen and molds, ventilation becomes inadequate to handle the excess moisture that daily activities produce.

Older homes, more likely built without vapor barriers, are vulnerable to moisture in the air. When moist, warm, indoor air touches cold surfaces inside the wall, it causes condensation.

A vapor barrier (plastic sheeting or foil) on the warm side of the wall keeps heated, moist indoor air from meeting cold surfaces inside the wall and causing condensation. This condensation makes insulation less effective and can result in peeling exterior paint.

Crawl spaces should be ventilated and covered with plastic sheeting to prevent mold spores in the moist ground from entering your house. Be on the alert for the musty odor that indicates mildew caused by water seepage.

APPLIANCES

Appliances that release combustion pollutlants are space heaters, gas ranges, ovens, furnaces, gas water heaters, gas clothes dryers, charcoal grills, wood or coal-burning stoves, and fireplaces. Combustion pollutants are particles or gases that result from burning fuels like gas, kerosene, wood, or coal. Combustion also releases water vapor that can cause high humidity, encouraging house dust mites, molds, and bacteria.

OTHER SOURCES OF MOLD

Other sources of mold in your home are kapok, foam pillows, wallpaper, dirty upholstery, old carpet padding, and wet wallpaper, foam pillows, dirty upholstery, and wet swimsuits and towels that have been thrown down on the floor rather than hung up to dry.

Don't forget to clean your home's gutters and downspouts and keep roofing in good repair, especially on the shady side of the house.

Asthma Resources Directory

Home Environment

Wet swimsuits and towels that have been thrown on the floor rather than hung up to dry are prime sources of mold.

Remember that dehumidifiers, cold mist vaporizers, humidifiers, and air conditioners must be kept clean because molds and bacteria will grow in their water

reservoirs. Fix water leaks promptly to avoid mold formation.

If you are building a home, there are techniques that may be employed to cut down on moisture, especially in basements. Be sure to talk to your architect or builder about placing sheet plastic barriers, especially for cement flooring, to act as moisture barriers.

DON'T FORGET YOUR CAR

Like your heating furnace, when you first turn on your car's air conditioner for the summer, it will throw out a spume of dust. Have the conditioner and the vents cleaned before you use the system. Remove the condensation water to keep the system free of mold.

Keep the floor mats clean and dry them in the sun. Don't allow children to eat or drink in the car and be very careful yourself. Spills on upholstery can support mold growth.

MOLD CONTROL — OUTDOOR MOLDS

Grass and leaves have a great deal of mold growth. When you rake, you scatter the mold and their spores become airborne. If you are allergic and you must care for your garden, wear a mask with an appropriate level of protection, and take your medication before gardening.

Do be sure your allergic children remain indoors while you are raking or mowing. Mold-allergic children shouldn't bounce on your leaf piles or walk through fallen leaves because that also disturbs the mold spores.

Mold-allergic children shouldn't bounce on your leaf piles or walk through fallen leaves because that disturbs the mold spores.

Keep your yard clean and don't use compost piles. Cut grass, barns, and wooded areas are sources of mold. Your compost heap is a major source of mold from decaying leaves and grass. Try to keep the garden clear of debris and

Allergy Products Directory
Copyrighted. Reproduction Prohibited by Law. 1259 El Camino #254, Menlo Park, CA 94025

Asthma Resources Directory
Home Environment

dying plants. Areas with hay stacks and barns or granaries and farms are important mold sources.

Garbage containers are mold sources as well and should be kept clean along with the area around them. Some sources recommend that borax be poured inside the cans to fight mold.

Garbage containers are mold sources and should be kept clean along with the area around them

---

Being outdoors on dry windy days, especially in rural areas, should be avoided. If farming or gardening activity is on-going, and children are very sensitive, they should stay in a clean-air room with the doors and windows closed.

Outdoor molds easily enter your home environment. Keep your windows closed and use a window air conditioner. If you can afford only one air conditioner, put it in the bedroom.

ANIMAL EXPOSURE
DANDER AS A CARRIER OF GLANDULAR SECRETIONS

Although your pet's dander or skin flakes are an allergic component of house dust, they are also an allergen by themselves. Dander is a long-lasting problem. It can remain in a home that has not had a pet for months, even years.

Some individuals are more sensitive to animal dander than others. Completely eliminating the animal from the home may be the only solution. For some, keeping the pets outdoors may be sufficient. However, children may actually spend more time outdoors with their pets because they are lonely for them.

GLANDULAR SECRETIONS

Dander carries glandular secretions that are on the skinflakes, the hair, or in saliva. Proteins from glandular secretion are carried on your pet's dander. When your pet licks itself, glandular secretions are spread over its fur.

Cat glandular secretion is such a strong allergen that you may have difficulty being with a friend who owns a cat. Your friend's clothing may have cat dander on it and you can react to the glandular secretion proteins carried by dander on the clothing.

33

Asthma Resources Directory

Home Environment

Cat glandular secretion is such a strong allergen, that you may have difficulty being with a friend who owns a cat.

Fel d **I**, a protein in cat skin, can be washed away. Some recent studies seem to indicate that *if* the cat is washed once a week for 10 minutes and *if* it spends most of its time outdoors, *if* the carpeting in the home is eliminated, and *if* air filters are used and *if* a thorough house cleaning schedule initiated, *then—some* time may be able to be spent with the cat.

These are severe measures for a possible occurrence, especially considering the pollen and moldy leaves that cling to your cat's fur. Also consider how you plan to bathe a cat once a week for 10 minutes. Further, these measures do not account for cat saliva, another strong allergen.

SALIVA AS A CARRIER

Pet saliva is an allergen. If you are very sensitive, your skin may turn red and itch where your pet licks you. Cat saliva deposited on cat hair during grooming aerosolizes and is found in the air, on your furniture and on your clothing. Saliva is also a carrier of gland secretion, picked up as cats lick themselves.

URINE

Sand boxes may become contaminted with cat urine and feces even when you don't own a cat. Be sure to keep sand boxes covered. As cats urinate, the urine becomes contaminated by the secretions that are on the skinflakes and the hair. Cat boxes are also sources of allergen from urine.

FLEAS

The majority of the fleas that your pet has been supporting remain in your home in the carpeting, in the cracks of the floor, or on furniture. Without your pet, it takes time and lots of it before that population actually declines.

Fleas can remain in their pupa stage for up to one year.

Keep this in mind when moving into a home where a pet once lived.

Fleas can remain in their pupa stage for up to one year. Keep this in mind when moving into a home where a pet once lived. (Bio-Integral Resource Center has a booklet,

Asthma Resources Directory

Home Environment

Least-Toxic Pest Management for Fleas PO Box 7414, Berkeley, CA 94704)

TRANSPORT

When your pet comes indoors, it brings moldy leaves clinging to its fur along with pollen it has picked up while romping. This increases the allergic load in the household. Even allowing a pet indoors for a short time is questionable because your forced air heating system can spread dander throughout the house. Once a pet is in a house, the allergen can remain in the environment for months; therefore, many doctors prefer that pets be given to other homes.

AVOIDANCE

Even when the decision to give a pet away is carried out, contacts with animal dander are difficult to avoid. Direct exposures can occur at a friend's home, a baby sitter's home, the park, a dog straying onto school property.

Dander travels on people's clothing and your child can be exposed to pet owners at school, at the supermarket, at a department store, on the street, at a friend's home (even when the friend does not own a dog), almost anywhere. Other family members may be in situations where there are animals and bring dander home on their clothing.

Allergy Products Directory
Copyrighted. Reproduction Prohibited by Law. 1259 El Camino #254, Menlo Park, CA 94025

Asthma Resources Directory
Environmental Irritants

ENVIRONMENTAL IRRITANTS

No matter how a product is formulated, there is the potential that someone can react to it. All a manufacturer can do is try to remove as many known irritants as possible.

Remember, even products marked unscented probably have scents known as masking scents.

The importance of any single source of pollution depends on how much pollutant it emits and how hazardous that emission is. It is important to maintain and adjust equipment properly to control emissions and use it in a well-ventilated area.

HOUSEHOLD IRRITANTS

Some sources like building materials, furnishings, and household products like air fresheners release pollutants just about all the time.

Other sources related pollutants intermittently: smoking, poorly vented or malfunctioning stoves, furnaces, or space heaters; using solvents while cleaning or hobby activities, paint strippers when redecorating; use of cleaning products. Sometimes pollutant concentrations can remain in the home for long periods after these activities.

Homes need to "leak" or allow an exchange of stale, indoor air with fresh outdoor air.

Homes need to "leak" or allow an exchange of stale, indoor air with fresh, outdoor air. The more airtight homes are (and newer ones are very airtight) the more you need to depend on ventilation systems to keep pollutant levels down.

Many substances in the environment can cause problems for sensitive individuals. Most of these are proteins, which can sensitize such as house dust mite, cockroach, and mold. Chemicals, like cleaning agents and bug killers, are usually irritants, but they can also be allergens.

Allergy Products Directory
Copyrighted. Reproduction Prohibited by Law. 1259 El Camino #254, Menlo Park, CA 94025

Asthma Resources Directory
Environmental Irritants

APARTMENTS AND OFFICE BUILDINGS

Apartments and office buildings have indoor air problems similar to homes because of furnishings, equipment, building materials, and cleaning products.

They have other problems caused by emissions from copiers and laser printers and ventilation controls designed to cut down on expenses. Newer buildings are very airtight and most do not allow for window opening. Facilities are cleaned nightly with strong products are used. During the day, multiple pollutant sources are at work.

Solutions here require eliminating or controlling sources of pollution, increasing ventilation, installing air cleaning devices.

THREE BASICS FOR CONTROLLING IRRITANTS AND ALLERGENS

Medication is not always helpful because as exposure continues, your sensitivity may increase and you may require more and more medication or your medication may stop working. So, the question becomes, what *can* you do?

1. CONTROL THE SOURCE

If you can eliminate a source of pollution or reduce its emissions, you've made an effective change in pollution level. Controlling the source of the pollution is the most effective solution.

Sources that contain asbestos can be sealed or enclosed; gas stoves can be adjusted; appliances can be vented outside. Generally, good maintenance can solve many problems.

Activities like painting, kerosene heating, cooking, welding, and soldering temporarily cause a higher pollution level. You should prepare for these by increasing ventilation in the area or by working outdoors if possible.

2. IMPROVE VENTILATION

Most home heating and air conditioning systems do not bring fresh air into the house. Newer homes are very airtight, only allowing low levels of fresh air exchange. Air-to-air heat exchangers are energy-efficient heat recovery ventilators that bring outdoor air into the home after warming it with outgoing, warm house air.

Asthma Resources Directory

Environmental Irritants

If you can, open a window or door or use a window or attic fan. Air conditioners can help as well. When using lavatory or kitchen facilities, use the fan.

3. USE AIR CLEANERS

Air cleaners, discussed in-depth in, *Controlling Your Environment: Improving Air Quality in Your Home,* are generally not effective in removing gaseous pollutants. They can be very effective particle removers, but how long they remain effective depends on how well you maintain them. Follow manufacturers instructions for maintenance and replacement.

WHAT ARE THE SOURCES OF IRRITANTS?

The following sources discuss various pollutants found in homes that can effect your health. Information indicating at what levels of pollution health effects will occur is limited. Most of us live in our homes without apparent problems. However, for those with sensitivities or other health problems, pollutant tolerance levels are lower.

SMOKING

Environmental tobacco smoke is considered a major indoor contaminant. The problem lies in the smoke rising from the burning end of a cigarette, pipe, or cigar and from exhaled smoke. More than 40 of the compounds in exhaled smoke are known to cause cancer and other compounds are strong irritants.

This environmental tobacco smoke is also called secondhand smoke and exposure to it is called passive smoking.

WHAT CAN YOU DO?

Do not allow smoking in your home. Avoid whenever possible being in enclosed environments with smokers. Be sure that your children are not exposed to environmental smoke in day care, baby sitting, play, or extra-curricular activities. See the chapter on *Smoking* for a more comprehensive discussion of this problem.

Asthma Resources Directory
Environmental Irritants

ALLERGIC AND BIOLOGICAL CONTAMINANTS

These contaminants are the molds, mildew, animal dander, and saliva proteins, house dust mites, pollen, and cockroaches that swirl through your home environment.

Sources are plants, people, animals, soil, plant debris, pets, mice, central air handling systems, and humidifiers.

Some biological contaminants cause allergic reactions such as hypersensitivity pneumonitis, allergic rhinitis, and some types of asthma. Symptoms of these contaminants are sneezing, watery eyes, coughing, shortness of breath, dizziness, lethargy, and fever.

WHAT CAN YOU DO?

If you can control the relative humidity level in your home, you can somewhat control the growth of some of these contaminants.

Air cleaners, air conditioners, and air filters are of help. The chapter on *Controlling Your Environment: Your Home Environment* gives specific steps you can take to lower the contaminant levels of your home.

Exhaust fans vented outdoors in your kitchen and bathroom eliminate the moisture that supports mold, mildew, and bacteria.

Try for a 30 to 50 percent relative humidity level. If you use a humidifier, keep it scrupulously clean to prevent bacteria and mold growth. Also, clean evaporation trays in air conditioners, dehumidifiers and refrigerators frequently.

Install and use exhaust fans vented outdoors in your kitchen and bathroom, and vent clothes dryers outdoors. There are two benefits to this. First, these fans and vents eliminate the moisture that supports mold, mildew, and bacterial growth. Second, these fans can reduce the levels of organic pollutants that vaporize from hot water.

Hotel non-smoking rooms may still allow pets.

Normal hotel cleaning does not clear a room of pet dander.

Ventilate attic and crawl spaces. If there is a leak or spill on a carpet, clean and dry (with fans, if necessary) the carpeting and underlying pad as quickly as possible to prevent mold growth.

Eliminating animals from your home further decreases contaminant levels

Asthma Resources Directory

Environmental Irritants

Hotel chains have varying policies on pets in their rooms. You may have a non-smoking room and yet be in a room that allows pets. Check with the hotel before making a reservation. Dander is a difficult substance to clear from a room, and normal hotel cleaning, no matter how thorough, cannot clear a room of pet dander.

IRRITANTS THAT INCITE OR AGGRAVATE ASTHMA

If you have asthma, your lungs are very reactive. Some inhalants may irritate you and cause bronchoconstriction and ongoing airway inflammation. Fumes, from perfumes, cosmetics, (or flowers) may cause problems.

These inhalant particles are extremely small and are less likely to be cleared from a room using a mechanical air purifier. Irritants like perfume, spray deodorant hair spray, air fresheners, cosmetics can cause allergic reactions, non-allergic reactions, or irritation.

WHAT CAN YOU DO?

Electrostatic precipitators and HEPA filters (ozone-free) can generally handle these particles that are smaller than pollen and are unlikely to be cleared from a room using a mechanical air purifier.

Try to eliminate the source of the irritant. Do not use perfumes and personal care items that cause you to react.

A SAMPLING OF PROBLEMS IN THE WORK PLACE

PAPAIN

an enzyme used in brewing beer and in formulating meat tenderizers, can cause immediate asthmatic symptoms

ANIMAL DANDERS

are a problem for veterinarians and lab workers, farmers, jockeys, and others who work around animals. Animal saliva and urine are also problems.

PROTEIN SECRETIONS

from birds have caused asthma and other problems for bird breeders.

FOOD

contaminants like insects or mold and even an allergy to wheat flour can cause asthma. People working as food

Asthma Resources Directory

Environmental Irritants

processors have developed sensitivity to green coffee beans, tea, garlic, and soybeans.

CASTOR BEANS

in fertilizer can cause asthma in workers and also in those living in the area.

SAWDUSTS

can cause asthma in workers.

TEXTILES

like cotton, hemp, and flax can cause asthma.

ANTIBIOTICS

can cause asthma in industry workers.

PLATINUM AND NICKEL

can sensitize workers and welders.

FORMALDEHYDE

is an irritant that can cause various problems both in those working in manufacturing and in those using the finished products.

POLYVINYL CHLORIDE

is the film that wraps meat and some individuals react when the film is heated for wrapping.

MOLDY HAY

can cause farmer's lung.

MALT WORKER'S DISEASE

from fungus spores.

WOOD-PULP WORKER'S DISEASE

from moldy logs.

According to Dr. Leslie Grammer, management consists of controlling exposure: changing jobs or retraining, moving from the area, ventilating efficiently, extracting dust and vapor efficiently.

Even if exposure levels are below legal limits, immunologic reactions may still occur.

Even if exposure levels are below legal limits, immunologic reactions may still occur. The goal should be prevention by improving ventilation and appropriate equipment, being aware of threshold limits, and education.

Asthma Resources Directory

Environmental Irritants

STOVES, FIREPLACES, HEATERS

Combustion products are produced indoors by unvented gas space heaters, gas ranges, ovens, furnaces, gas water heaters, gas clothes dryers, charcoal grills, wood, gas, or coal-burning stoves, and fireplaces, improperly installed or maintained chimneys and flues, and from cracks in heat exchangers.

How much pollutant is released depends on the type of appliance, the fuel it uses, its installation, maintenance, and ventilation. Are vents and chimneys inspected?

Combustion releases water vapor that can cause high humidity, encouraging house dust mites, molds, and bacteria.

The combustion pollutants are particles or gases that result from burning fuels like gas, kerosene, wood, or coal in various appliances. These products of combustion are carbon monoxide, nitrogen dioxide, particles, sulfur dioxide, unburned hydrocarbons, and aldehydes.

These gases can cause discomfort or illness even if you are healthy. Effects can range from headache and breathing difficulties to death from the carbon monoxide of faulty heaters. Effects may be immediate or become apparent after long exposure. Effects depend on age and health.

If you have asthma or respiratory disease, this type of exposure is particularly damaging. Further, combustion also releases water vapor that can cause high humidity, encouraging house dust mites, molds, and bacteria.

WHAT CAN YOU DO?

VENT OUTDOORS

Appliances should be vented outdoors to prevent the noxious by-products of combustion from flowing throughout your living and working areas. Be sure all pilot lights burn blue, a sign of cleaner, complete combustion; a yellow flame indicates a need for adjustment.

BUY SAFE HEATERS AND APPLIANCES

Oil heaters should have a UL label. Gas appliances should have an AGA or UL label.

IMPROVE INDOOR VENTILATION

If you must use unvented kerosene or gas space heaters, follow instructions very carefully. Be sure all pilot lights

Asthma Resources Directory
Environmental Irritants

burn blue. Keep a safety screen around any appliances with an open flame. Keep the door opened and open a window.

USE FUEL APPROPRIATELY

Use only the correct fuel for each appliance. Never try to increase a fire with kerosene or gasoline. When you must refill an oil or kerosene unit, don't overfill it. The oil expands as it warms and can flood the burner. Do not fill the heater while it is burning. Store fuels outside of the house in the correct containers.

INSTALL HOODS

Install stove hoods with fans vented outdoors. If you can't install a hood in your kitchen, use an exhaust fan. Do not use a gas stove for heat. If you are purchasing a new gas stove, consider one with a pilotless ignition, called an electronic ignition.

USE WOODSTOVES SAFELY

Your woodstove should be air tight and meet EPA emission standards. Use aged wood and follow manufacturer's instructions. Look for asbestos-free replacement gaskets made of fiberglass. Inspect chimneys and keep them clean.

KEEP CENTRAL AIR SYSTEM IN REPAIR

Have a professional inspect your central air handling systems and repair any damage. Check to see that your gas heater has a safety shut-off.

For more information, call your local American Lung Association in the white pages of the phone book.

HOUSEHOLD PRODUCTS

Remember that we use many chemicals on a daily basis: cleaning, disinfecting, cosmetic, and hobby products. For safety reasons, store these items in well ventilated areas out of the reach of children and, preferably, in locked cabinets.

WHAT CAN YOU DO?

Work in well-ventilated areas, or open a door and windows, or work outdoors. Safely dispose of old containers, unneeded containers, or containers that are almost empty. Buy only quantities that you need for the project at hand. Read and follow all health hazard

43

Asthma Resources Directory

Environmental Irritants

information and precautions. Dress in work clothes that can be removed when the job is done. Wear an appropriate mask.

Professional dry cleaners use perchloroethylene which can be inhaled from clothing that has been dry cleaned. Do not accept clothing with a strong smell. It should have been properly dried by the cleaner. Request that this be done.

FORMALDEHYDE

Formaldehyde is used in building materials and household products. It is also a by-product of combustion from unvented gas stoves or kerosene space heaters.

Formaldehyde is used in permanent press clothing and drapes, in glues and adhesives and in some paints. If your home has furniture or cabinets made from pressed wood that use urea-formaldehyde adhesives, those products will

---

Formaldehyde is used in building materials and household products.

It is also a by-product of combustion from unvented gas stoves or kerosene space heaters.

---

emit formaldehyde. These products are: particleboard (subflooring and shelving), hardwood plywood paneling, fiberboard (drawer fronts, cabinets, furniture tops). Other sources of formaldehyde are: carpeting, paper goods, household cleaners, and water repellents.

In the 1970's, urea-formaldehyde foam insulation was installed in many homes as added insulation, resulting in high indoor concentrations of formaldehyde. This problem was reported on and followed by American Allergy Association since many symptom complaints had been received.

In March, 1980, the National Academy of Sciences concluded that formaldehyde did pose a serious health problem "even at extremely low airborne concentrations"

Formaldehyde vaporizes at low temperatures. Off-gassing releases vapors that can cause a variety of symptoms. In March, 1980, the National Academy of Sciences concluded that formaldehyde did pose a serious health problem: "even at extremely low airborne concnentrations" it will irritate the eyes, nose, and throat of some individuals. The quantity of formaldehyde emission

Allergy Products Directory
Copyrighted. Reproduction Prohibited by Law. 1259 El Camino #254, Menlo Park, CA 94025

Asthma Resources Directory
Environmental Irritants

decreases with age of product, lower temperatures, and humidity.

Since 1985, the Department of Housing and Urban Development (HUD) has restricted plywood and particle board for mobile homes only to those materials that conform to specific formaldehyde emission limits.

WHAT CAN YOU DO?

Ask about formaldehyde content of pressed wood products, building materials, and furniture before buying. There is a possibility that coating pressed wood products with polyurethane may reduce emissions for some length of time, but every surface area, including edges must be covered. You may also want to investigate the possibility of covering the cabinets with Formica®. Try to keep heat and humidity levels down.

INDOOR PLANTS

Not all sources of pollution are chemical or high-tech. Indoor plants in home or office are a source of mold. Large plants with large leaves can become dust collectors. Their leaves need regular cleaning. If you have enough plants, misting them will raise humidity levels somewhat and watering them will cause carpet damage and mold from water spills.

WHAT CAN YOU DO?

Don't over-water houseplants because you will encourage mold and microorganism growth on the soil. If you are sensitive to mold, don't have house plants, especially in your bedroom. Mold can even grow on the sides of the pots.

The notion that houseplants can help improve air quality because of their oxygen output is subject to disussion. We've heard said that it would take a greenhouse worth of plants to supply sufficient oxygen – but then we'd have a greenhouse worth of mold and very high humidity levels to pamper house dust mites.

PESTICIDES

We use pesticides at home to kill insects, termites, and as disinfectants. We also use them on the lawn and garden. These products are sold as sprays, powders, crystals,

Asthma Resources Directory

Environmental Irritants

liquids, balls, and foggers. It is easy to track these around the house and children are major victims of pesticide poisonings.

Symptoms are irritation to your eyes, nose and throat. Higher exposures to certain insecticides have caused various symptoms: headache and nausea.

> EPA has concern that exposure to cyclodienes might cause long-term liver damage and central nervous system damage. For these reasons, cyclodienes are not permitted to be sold any longer; neither are chlordane, aldrin, dieldrin, and heptachlor. If you have any products so labeled, dispose of them immediately and safely.

WHAT CAN YOU DO?

When you garden, try wearing clothes and shoes that you use only for gardening. When you finish, take your shoes off and put them away somewhere outside the main house. Take your clothes and socks off immediately to be washed so that pesticide residues are not brought indoors.

Follow manufacturer's instructions. If you must dilute a product, do it outdoors. Apply it according to directions and don't over use. If you must use products like these indoors, open doors and windows. If you must spray house plants or pets, do so outdoors.

Do not buy more than you need.

It is better to use and then dispose of these products safely, according to their directions.

Do not store these products in your home. Do not store them within reach of children. Keep these products in locked, ventilated cabinets. Do not buy more than you need. It is better to use and then dispose of these products safely, according to their directions.

National Pesticides Telecommunications Network, 800-858-PEST (7378), in Texas, 806-743-3091, 8:00 am to 6 pm central time, provides information about pesticides and pesticide exposure to the public and to physicians.

ASBESTOS

Asbestos becomes a problem when it begins to deteriorate or is damaged in some way. It is found in insulation, acoustic materials, floor tiles, and the door

Asthma Resources Directory
Environmental Irritants

gaskets of wood-burning stoves. Older homes are more likely to have asbestos in furnace insulation, shingles, millboard, textured paints, and floor tiles.

Fibers in the air are inhaled and can cause cancers or scarring of the lungs years after exposure. Fibers from exposures outside the home can cling to clothing and be brought home.

WHAT CAN YOU DO?

If asbestos is not damaged or crumbling, EPA recommends that it is best to leave it alone. Don't start projects requiring any abrasion of asbestos. Such projects will release fibers into the air. Only qualified contractors should be used to remove asbestos or to handle it in any way.

EPA has an assistance line: 202-554-1404. Call it to find out if your state has a training and certification program for asbestos removal contractors.

LEAD

Lead-based paint is a common pollutant source in older home. Exposure can result in serious problelms: lethargy, kidney, nervous system, and blood cell problems, coma, and convulsions. Children effected by lead can show mental and physical developmental delays, lower IQ levels, decreased attention spans, and behavioral problems. A developing fetus can be seriously harmed.

WHAT CAN YOU DO?

Keep play areas as clean as you can. Pay special attention to window sills and ledges, cribs, banisters, any painted surface. Wash them with a solution of high phosphate, powdered, automatic dishwasher detergent and warm water. (Be sure to protect your hands.) Keep toys and stuffed animals washed. Wash children's hands before they eat, before they go to bed, and as soon as they come inside after playing outdoors.

Do not burn painted wood since the paint may be leaded.

Do not sand or scrape lead paint because you can inhale particles.

Do not burn painted wood since the paint may be leaded. Do not sand or scrape lead paint because you can inhale the particles. If any work needs to be done involving

Asthma Resources Directory

Environmental Irritants

the removal or sanding of lead paint, keep away from the premises until the work is finished and the area is clean.

For help in finding an agency that can test for lead, try your state's department of health or housing department. You'll need someone trained to remove lead-based paints.

Another method requiring a professional is encapsulation in which a film is sprays over the lead-

If you work in construction, demolition, in a radiator repair shop, or use lead in your hobby, you may be bringing it home on your hands and on your clothing.

painted walls. The film is cured and a finish coat put over it. This finish coat can then be painted.

If you work in construction, in demolition, in a radiator repair shop, or use lead in your hobby, you may be bringing it home on your hands and on your clothing. The best defense is to change your clothes before you go home. Wash these clothes separately.

OTHER CHEMICALS

Many chemicals can irritate the lungs and cause wheezing. Chemicals that are generally considered irritants are ammonia, chlorine, formaldehyde, hydrogen chloride, nitrous oxide, ozone, phosgene, sulphur dioxide, and toluene in dyes can also cause irritation. Strong odors like aerosol sprays, perfumes, cleansers, and room fresheners can also be problems.

At home, avoidance is the main control; containment of the odor, if possible or a high-efficiency filtration system.

ODORS

Your negative response to an odor depends on how your trigeminal nerve perceives the odor as an irritant. Most people react negatively to irritating smells like ammonia but allergic individuals may wheeze or have drippy noses or hives as a response to odors that don't bother other people. (See "The role of odors and vapors in allergic disease" by A. J. Horesh in the *Journal of Asthma Research* 4:125, 1966 for a comprehensive listing of indoor odors.)

Allergic individuals may wheeze or have drippy noses or hives as a response to odors that don't bother other people.

Asthma Resources Directory

Environmental Irritants

At home, irritants can be strong odors like perfumes, room fresheners, cleansers, deodorant sprays, and aerosol sprays. Some mattress and pillow encasings used for house dust mite control have a very strong odor. Mothballs and flakes, kerosene fumes, insecticide sprays, floor wax, newly printed newspapers, cleaners with chlorine and ammonia, brass polishers, tobacco smoke are all examples of fumes that can make allergic rhinitis or asthma worse.

While driving, be aware that fumes in heavy traffic, particularly in states or coutries without smog control devices on cars can be highly irritating. Driving in tunnels and in cities or being stuck in traffic can provoke symptoms.

At home, irritants can be strong odors like room fresheners, deodorant sprays, and aerosol sprays.

The odors of certain foods being fried can cause problems for sensitive individuals, while burning wood and kerosene used for heating produce particulates and fumes.

Do it yourselfers run into difficulties with paints, paint cleaners, paint thinners, paint removers, varnishes.

Odors are hard enough to avoid when you know about the source. When they come upon you unaware, they are more difficult to cope with. For some time now, magazines have been produced with scent strips in advertisements. Department store bills can also arrive with scent-saturated adds.

Department store bills can arrive with scent-saturated strips.

The strips either have a scratch strip or are sealed in a packet. Both the scratch strip and the packet are supposed to keep the odor controlled until either the strip is scratched or the packet is opened to release the smell.

Unfortunately, the scents are so powerful that the odor is strongly obvious as soon as the magazine or envelope arrives. Reactions to these strong odors range from stinging eyes to tearing or headache.

WHAT CAN YOU DO?

The prime source of relief is to avoid odors. Do not use perfumes and air fresheners. Avoid products with smells that irritate you and look for alternatives.

Avoidance is not always within your power. You cannot control the perfume worn by the stranger who sits beside

Asthma Resources Directory

Environmental Irritants

you on a bus, but you can move. You need not prepare certain foods. You can sit in non-smoking sections. You can tell your friends not to smoke when they are with you or at your home. Smoke odor is very difficult to eradicate from drapes, carpets, and upholstered furniture.

If you can't avoid frying foods that cause problems, turn on the vents and open windows and doors. If you are not doing the frying, leave.

Products with strong smells should be safely stored outside and away from the house. If you find that your new mattress encasing has an objectionable odor, air it outside until the odor is no longer a problem.

---

*Air out carpeting in your garage or some sheltered area
before installation.*

Air out carpeting in your garage or some sheltered area before installation. New furniture and any new building materials may need airing. When bringing these new items inside, be sure doors and windows are opened.

Avoid traveling during rush hour if possible. If that is unavoidable, keep your car windows closed. Use a car air conditioner that recirculates inner air. Keep your windows closed during pollen season. Try covering the car's air vents with cheese cloth when operating the air conditioner to trap some of the mold growth in the system.

Try not to exercise when air pollution levels are high. Don't exercise near heavily used roads, especially if traffic is stalled.

Problems with the strong smells that permeate a magazine or bill because of enclosed advertising scent strips are more difficult to handle because the problem comes to you. You have to pay the bill or you want to read the magazine.

---

*Some magazines companies are able to identify a subscriber
and eliminate the scent strip
because their computer system is sophisticated.*

(Writer's Note: The fragrance was still strong through the plastic wrap of a magazine that arrived at our home over eight months ago and left un opened as a test.)

Write to the publisher and request elimination of the strips from your magazines. Write to the department store and request that strips be eliminated from your bills or that a warning be printed on the envelope of the bill so someone

Asthma Resources Directory

Environmental Irritants

else can open and respond to it. Request that packaging be used that does not allow odor to escape until opened.

Some magazines companies are responsive to complaints from individual consumers because they are able to identify a particular subscriber and eliminate the scent strip from that particular magazine because of the sophistication of the computer systems they use. Others find the cost of such action extremely costly.

If there is no result in relief, state that you are canceling your subscription after many years of readership. Then say exactly why you are doing so. Write the advertiser to say that you will not buy the product and clearly state why.

If the problem is with department store bills and your request has not gotten results, you can cancel your account and clearly state why.

We urge everyone who has to contend with scent-strips to speak up. As more of us speak up, we will be heard.

CARS

Some makes of cars pull outside air in through their air conditioning systems. Although an advantage in clean air situations, these car air conditioners can be a problem when driving in heavy traffic or behind cars with particularly dirty exhausts because the air conditioning system can draw the fumes into your car. Exhaust fumes from your car can enter your home from an attached garage.

WHAT CAN YOU DO?

If possible, try not to drive during rush hours when traffic is heavy. If unavoidable, keep the car windows closed. Select a car that recirculates car air through the conditioning system or discuss a car filter with your doctor. Also ask about mold control services through Ford and General Motors dealers.

A garage that is attached to your home should treated as part of your home. Never run the car's engine with the garage door closed or with the connecting door to your home opened.

In fact, be safe. Don't run the car inside the garage at all. If you must make repairs, pull the car outside. Fumes from the car's exhaust can enter your home even with the connecting door closed.

Asthma Resources Directory

Environmental Irritants

For some of the information in this article we are indebted to

American Lung Assn.
US Consumer Product Safety Commission
US Environmental Protection Agency

HOUSE HOLD CLEANING TIPS:

Although we've collected these cleaning tips over the years from a variety of sources, we cannot vouch for them because individuals have differing needs and requirements. Remember, some of these approaches will be more effective than others and most of them require a great deal of elbow grease.

We're always looking for more tips, so write and tell us what you've discovered.

1. Clean brass with a mixture of equal parts of salt and flour and a few drops of vinegar. Or squeeze lemon juice on a soft cloth and apply; rinse off with warm water and dry. Or apply a cut lemon directly.

2. Clean copper with a squeeze of lemon juice on a soft cloth and apply; rinse off with warm water and dry.

3. Clean silver with baking soda and water and rub. Or 1 tsp salt and 1 tbsp baking soda to one quart of water; boil for 3 minutes in an aluminum pan or pot lined with aluminum foil; use with a soft cloth

4. Clean plastic laminate cabinets with club soda

5. Garbage Can Mold, Bacteria: pour some borax inside the can

6. Air Fresheners: baking soda is a good odor absorbent

7. Tile and Glass Cleaners: clean with baking soda on a dampened cloth and rinse

8. Lubricants: use castor oil instead of oil lubricants. Check with the manufacturer first, since you don't want to damage the motor.

9. Ammonia-based Cleaner: substitute vinegar, salt, water

10. Furniture Polish: lemon juice with twice as much vegetable oil or 3 parts olive oil and 1 part white vinegar.

11. Drain Cleaner: boiling water with 1/4 cup baking soda and 1/4 cup vinegar plus a plunger.

Allergy Products Directory
Copyrighted. Reproduction Prohibited by Law. 1259 El Camino #254, Menlo Park, CA 94025

Asthma Resources Directory

Household Maintenance

HOUSEHOLD MAINTENANCE

This chapter presents a selection of cleaning and repair products that may be less likely to irritate lungs and skin. As always, what works for someone else may not work for you and what does not irritate you may not do quite the job you envision.

CLEANING AIDS

AFM SafeChoice Carpet Shampoo

Dye-free, odorless; do not use on wool carpeting
Available from:
Allergy Resources
Mail: PO Box 888 (APD)
UPS: 264 Brookridge Ave. (APD)
Palmer Lake, CO 80133
Orders 800-USE-FLAX (873-3529)
Company plans a move; use 800 #
and:
Allergy-Asthma Shopper™
PO Box 239 (APD)
Fate, TX 75132
800-447-1100
Fax 903-883-4513

AFM Super Clean

Odor-free, dye-free all-purpose cleaner for grease, dirt, oil, film; use on floors, woodwork, walls, countertops, tubs, tile, furniture, rugs, fabrics, laundry
Available from:
AFM Enterprises, Inc.
1960 Chicago E7 (APD)
Riverside, CA 92507
909-781-6860
909-781-6861
Fax 909-781-6892
and:
Allergy Relief Shop,™Inc.
3371 Whittle Springs Rd. (APD)
Knoxville, TN 37917
Orders 800-626-2810
Questions 615-522-2795
and:
Allergy Resources
Mail: PO Box 888 (APD)
UPS: 264 Brookridge Ave. (APD)

Palmer Lake, CO 80133
Orders 800-USE-FLAX (873-3529)
Company plans a move; use 800 #
and:
Allergy-Asthma Shopper™
PO Box 239 (APD)
Fate, TX 75132
800-447-1100
Fax 903-883-4513
and:
Flowright Int'l Products
1495 N.W. Gilman Blvd. #4 (APD)
Issaquah, WA 98027
206-392-8357
and:
N.E.E.D.S.
527 Charles Ave. 12A (APD)
Syracuse, NY 13209
800-634-1380
Fax 800-295-NEED (6333)

All Purpose Polish and Wax

Liquid or paste to clean and polish furniture, most floors and vinyl, and metal finishes on automobiles and applliances
Available from:
Allergy Relief Shop,™Inc.
3371 Whittle Springs Rd. (APD)
Knoxville, TN 37917
Orders 800-626-2810
Questions 615-522-2795
and:
Flowright Int'l Products
1495 N.W. Gilman Blvd. #4 (APD)
Issaquah, WA 98027
206-392-8357
and:
N.E.E.D.S.
527 Charles Ave. 12A (APD)
Syracuse, NY 13209

Asthma Resources Directory

Household Maintenance

800-634-1380
Fax 800-295-NEED (6333)

Allersearch X-Mite™ All-in-One

Controls dust mites, mite allergen, and animal dander; can be used on carpets and some fabrics; moist powder based on tannic acid; covers 115 sq. ft. of carpet
Available from:
American Allergy Supply
PO Box 722022 (APD)
Houston, TX 77272-2022
800-321-1096
713-995-6110
and:
National Allergy Supply, Inc.
4400 Georgia Hwy. 120 (APD)
PO Box 1658 (APD)
Duluth, GA 30136
800-522-1448
In Atlanta 404-623-8077
Fax 404-623-5568

Ar-Ex® Safe Suds

"Hypo-allergenic;" lanolin-free; unscented; soap-free
Available from:
Ar-Ex Ltd.
156 N. Jefferson St. #205 (APD)
Chicago, IL 60661
312-879-0017
Fax 312-879-0019

Arm & Hammer® Detergent

Detergent, perfume, and dye free
Available from
Supermarkets

Automatic Dish Washing Machine Detergent

Biodegradeable agent for removing oil, grease, and food products; spot-free
Available from:
Allergy Relief Shop,™Inc.
3371 Whittle Springs Rd. (APD)
Knoxville, TN 37917
Orders 800-626-2810
Questions 615-522-2795

Bissell® Carpet Care Allergen Control

Eliminates allergens in carpets and upholstery; suitable for non-cartridge carpet cleaners
Available from:
Priorities®
70 Walnut St. (APD)
Wellesley, MA 02181
800-553-5398

Capture® Carpet Care

Dry carpet cleaner; moisture-free use does not support mold growth; includes spot cleaner and brush
Available from:
Allergy Asthma Technology
4151 N. Kedzie (APD)
PO Box 18398 (APD)
Chicago, IL 60618
800-621-5545
312-465-8020
Fax 312-465-7619
and:
Allergy Control Products, Inc.
96 Danbury Rd. (APD)
PO Box 793 (APD)
Ridgefield, CT 06877
800-422-DUST (3878)
203-438-9580
Fax 203-431-8963

Carpet Shampoo

Use as cleaner; removes grease, dirt, oil films; any carpet cleaning equipment
Available from:
AFM Enterprises, Inc.
1960 Chicago E7 (APD)
Riverside, CA 92507
909-781-6860
909-781-6861
Fax 909-781-6892
and:
Allergy Relief Shop,™Inc.
3371 Whittle Springs Rd. (APD)
Knoxville, TN 37917
Orders 800-626-2810
Questions 615-522-2795
and:

Allergy Products Directory
Copyrighted. Reproduction Prohibited by Law. 1259 El Camino #254,Menlo Park, CA 94025

Asthma Resources Directory
Household Maintenance

Flowright Int'l Products
1495 N.W. Gilman Blvd. #4 (APD)
Issaquah, WA 98027
206-392-8357

Deodorizing Pouch
Fragrance-free zeolite in a 9"x9" mesh pouch adsorbs odors; for enclosed spaces, closets, basements, and cars; reusable, reactivates with sun exposure; company notes that there is minimal residual dust only upon opening seal
Available from:
Absolute Environmental's Allergy Store
2615 S. University Dr. (APD)
Davie, FL 33328
Nationwide 800-771-ACHOO (2246)
In FL 800-329-3773
Broward 305-472-3773
Fax 305-474-0133
and:
Allergy Resources
Mail: PO Box 888 (APD)
UPS: 264 Brookridge Ave. (APD)
Palmer Lake, CO 80133
Orders 800-USE-FLAX (873-3529)
Company plans a move; use 800 #
and:
Signatures
19465 Brennan Ave. (APD)
Perris, CA 92599
800-777-0327
909-943-2021

Dip-N-Glow
Jewelry cleaner
Available from:
Flowright Int'l Products
1495 N.W. Gilman Blvd. #4 (APD)
Issaquah, WA 98027
206-392-8357

Dishwashing Liquid
Color-free, fragrance-free, alcohol-free
Available from:
Janice Corp.
198 US Hwy. 46 (APD)
Budd Lake, NJ 07828-3001

800-JANICES (526-4237)
Fax 201-691-5459

DRI-APP™
Applicator for cleaning powders
Available from:
Allergy Control Products, Inc.
96 Danbury Rd. (APD)
PO Box 793 (APD)
Ridgefield, CT 06877
800-422-DUST (3878)
203-438-9580
Fax 203-431-8963

Dust Grabber™
Fabric with permanent electrostatic surface charge; washable; odor-free, chemical-free; does not feel tacky; leaves no film; 14x14 cloth stretchable, can be clipped to mop head
Available from:
National Allergy Supply, Inc.
4400 Georgia Hwy. 120 (APD)
PO Box 1658 (APD)
Duluth, GA 30136
800-522-1448
In Atlanta 404-623-8077
Fax 404-623-5568

E-Z-On Shoe Polish
Self-polishing, little or no buffing; no petroleum distillates; white, black, brown
Available from:
Flowright Int'l Products
1495 N.W. Gilman Blvd. #4 (APD)
Issaquah, WA 98027
206-392-8357

E.Z. Maid
Dish washing and all-purpose liquid; unscented; non-abrasive
Available from:
Allergy Resources
Mail: PO Box 888 (APD)
UPS: 264 Brookridge Ave. (APD)
Palmer Lake, CO 80133
Orders 800-USE-FLAX (873-3529)
Company plans a move; use 800 #

Asthma Resources Directory

Household Maintenance

and:
Flowright Int'l Products
1495 N.W. Gilman Blvd. #4 (APD)
Issaquah, WA 98027
206-392-8357

Ivory Snow®

Clinically proven to be mild to skin
Available from
Supermarkets

Laundry Detergent

Color-free, fragrance-free, alcohol-free
Available from:
Janice Corp.
198 US Hwy. 46 (APD)
Budd Lake, NJ 07828-3001
800-JANICES (526-4237)
Fax 201-691-5459

Libwipes

Edge sealed limited linting cotton for scratch-free wiping; does not attract air-borne particles with electrostatic charges; high absorbency
Available from:
Liberty Industries, Inc.
133 Commerce St. (APD)
E. Berlin, CT 06023
800-828-5656
In CT 828-6361
Fax 203-828-8879

Like Nu Rust Remover

Removes rust from metal and concrete surfaces; can remove water spots from tile
Available from:
Allergy Relief Shop,™ Inc.
3371 Whittle Springs Rd. (APD)
Knoxville, TN 37917
Orders 800-626-2810
Questions 615-522-2795
and:
Flowright Int'l Products
1495 N.W. Gilman Blvd. #4 (APD)
Issaquah, WA 98027
206-392-8357
and:

N.E.E.D.S.
527 Charles Ave. 12A (APD)
Syracuse, NY 13209
800-634-1380
Fax 800-295-NEED (6333)

Nature Clean All Purpose Cleaning Lotion

Free of fragrance; "hypo-allergenic"
Available from:
Allergy Shop, Ltd.
3420 Cardston Crescent N.W. (APD)
Calgary, AB T2L 0S6
Canada
403-289-9052

Nature Clean Window/Glass Cleaner

Free of ammonia, dyes, perfumes, chlorine bleach, enzymes
Available from:
Allergy Shop, Ltd.
3420 Cardston Crescent N.W. (APD)
Calgary, AB T2L 0S6
Canada
403-289-9052

Power Plus

Laundry concentrate; no fragrances
Available from:
Allergy Alternative
440 Godfrey Dr. (APD)
Windsor, CA 95492
800-838-1514
and:
Allergy Resources
Mail: PO Box 888 (APD)
UPS: 264 Brookridge Ave. (APD)
Palmer Lake, CO 80133
Orders 800-USE-FLAX (873-3529)
Company plans a move; use 800 #
and:
Flowright Int'l Products
1495 N.W. Gilman Blvd. #4 (APD)
Issaquah, WA 98027
206-392-8357
and:
N.E.E.D.S.
527 Charles Ave. 12A (APD)

Asthma Resources Directory
Household Maintenance

Syracuse, NY 13209
800-634-1380
Fax 800-295-NEED (6333)

Power Scrubber

Keeps hands out of gloves and away from soap and water; three rotating brushes (nylon, stainless steel sponge, bristle) clean pots and pans; water resistant; requires 3 C batteries
Available from:
Home Trends
1450 Lyell Ave. (APD)
Rochester, NY 14606-2184
716-254-6520
Fax 716-458-9245

Shingle Protek

Flame retardant for wood shingled roofs; water resistant
Available from:
Allergy Relief Shop,™ Inc.
3371 Whittle Springs Rd. (APD)
Knoxville, TN 37917
Orders 800-626-2810
Questions 615-522-2795
and:
Flowright Int'l Products
1495 N.W. Gilman Blvd. #4 (APD)
Issaquah, WA 98027
206-392-8357
and:
N.E.E.D.S.
527 Charles Ave. 12A (APD)
Syracuse, NY 13209
800-634-1380
Fax 800-295-NEED (6333)

Soft N' Fresh Fabric Softener

Fragrance-free; citrus-free
Available from:
Allergy Resources
Mail: PO Box 888 (APD)
UPS: 264 Brookridge Ave. (APD)
Palmer Lake, CO 80133
Orders 800-USE-FLAX (873-3529)
Company plans a move; use 800 #

Soil Away

Fabric stain remover for ink, blood, crayon, mud, lipstick; no synthetic fragrance or color
Available from:
Allergy Resources
Mail: PO Box 888 (APD)
UPS: 264 Brookridge Ave. (APD)
Palmer Lake, CO 80133
Orders 800-USE-FLAX (873-3529)
Company plans a move; use 800 #
and:
Flowright Int'l Products
1495 N.W. Gilman Blvd. #4 (APD)
Issaquah, WA 98027
206-392-8357
and:
N.E.E.D.S.
527 Charles Ave. 12A (APD)
Syracuse, NY 13209
800-634-1380
Fax 800-295-NEED (6333)

Spray Cleaner

Color-free, fragrance-free, alcohol-free
Available from:
Janice Corp.
198 US Hwy. 46 (APD)
Budd Lake, NJ 07828-3001
800-JANICES (526-4237)
Fax 201-691-5459

Super Clean

All-purpose cleaner without fumes; non-irritating to skin
Available from:
Allergy Resources
Mail: PO Box 888 (APD)
UPS: 264 Brookridge Ave. (APD)
Palmer Lake, CO 80133
Orders 800-USE-FLAX (873-3529)
Company plans a move; use 800 #
and:
N.E.E.D.S.
527 Charles Ave. 12A (APD)
Syracuse, NY 13209
800-634-1380
Fax 800-295-NEED (6333)
and:

Asthma Resources Directory

Household Maintenance

Priorities®
70 Walnut St. (APD)
Wellesley, MA 02181
800-553-5398

Twice as Gentle
Liquid detergent free of perfume, coloring, brighteners, emulsifiers, no strong alkalis, enzymes, phosphates, fillers
Available from
Boots Chemists, England

Ultra Safe
Air cleaner with vacuum attachment for computers, reading boxes; 350 CFM; filters 650 sq. ft.; filtered motor, intake has washable prefilter and exhaust chamber has prefilter, carbon filter; HEPA filter; blower; commercial use, stainles steel case, casters; 27"x25"x12"
Available from:
Allergy Relief Shop,™Inc.
3371 Whittle Springs Rd. (APD)
Knoxville, TN 37917
Orders 800-626-2810
Questions 615-522-2795
and:
AllerMed Corp.
31 Steel Rd. (APD)
Wylie, TX 75098
214-442-4898
Fax 214-442-4897

Woolworths Home Brand Laundry Soap
"Less irritating" laundry soap; available in local groceries and markets in Australia and New Zealand

Zeolite® Odor Neutralizer
Non-toxic, non allergenic powder attracts odors; fragrance-free; for carpets and upholstery
Available from:
Absolute Environmental's Allergy Store
2615 S. University Dr. (APD)
Davie, FL 33328
Nationwide 800-771-ACHOO (2246)

In FL 800-329-3773
Broward 305-472-3773
Fax 305-474-0133

REPAIRS AND MAINTENANCE AIDS

3 in 1 Adhesive
Odor-free, bonds ceramic, vinyl, and parquet tiles; use test application
Available from:
AFM Enterprises, Inc.
1960 Chicago E7 (APD)
Riverside, CA 92507
909-781-6860
909-781-6861
Fax 909-781-6892
and:
Allergy Relief Shop,™Inc.
3371 Whittle Springs Rd. (APD)
Knoxville, TN 37917
Orders 800-626-2810
Questions 615-522-2795
and:
Allergy Resources
Mail: PO Box 888 (APD)
UPS: 264 Brookridge Ave. (APD)
Palmer Lake, CO 80133
Orders 800-USE-FLAX (873-3529)
Company plans a move; use 800 #
and:
Flowright Int'l Products
1495 N.W. Gilman Blvd. #4 (APD)
Issaquah, WA 98027
206-392-8357
and:
N.E.E.D.S.
527 Charles Ave. 12A (APD)
Syracuse, NY 13209
800-634-1380
Fax 800-295-NEED (6333)

Acrylacq
Replaces lacquer; clear, high gloss for gym floors, stair railings, hardwood floors
Available from:
AFM Enterprises, Inc.
1960 Chicago E7 (APD)

58

Asthma Resources Directory

Household Maintenance

Riverside, CA 92507
909-781-6860
909-781-6861
Fax 909-781-6892
and:
Allergy Relief Shop,™Inc.
3371 Whittle Springs Rd. (APD)
Knoxville, TN 37917
Orders 800-626-2810
Questions 615-522-2795
and:
Flowright Int'l Products
1495 N.W. Gilman Blvd. #4 (APD)
Issaquah, WA 98027
206-392-8357
and:
N.E.E.D.S.
527 Charles Ave. 12A (APD)
Syracuse, NY 13209
800-634-1380
Fax 800-295-NEED (6333)

AFM Caulking Compound

Use as putty for windows, cracks, and repairs
Available from:
Flowright Int'l Products
1495 N.W. Gilman Blvd. #4 (APD)
Issaquah, WA 98027
206-392-8357
and:
N.E.E.D.S.
527 Charles Ave. 12A (APD)
Syracuse, NY 13209
800-634-1380
Fax 800-295-NEED (6333)

Almighty Adhesive

Bonds wood, plastic, marble, ceramic, some pavers, slate, metal, carpet, parquet, furniture, and cork
Available from:
AFM Enterprises, Inc.
1960 Chicago E7 (APD)
Riverside, CA 92507
909-781-6860
909-781-6861
Fax 909-781-6892
and:
Allergy Relief Shop,™Inc.

3371 Whittle Springs Rd. (APD)
Knoxville, TN 37917
Orders 800-626-2810
Questions 615-522-2795

Carpet Adhesive

For installing textiles and various carpet floor coverings
Available from:
Allergy Relief Shop,™Inc.
3371 Whittle Springs Rd. (APD)
Knoxville, TN 37917
Orders 800-626-2810
Questions 615-522-2795
and:
Flowright Int'l Products
1495 N.W. Gilman Blvd. #4 (APD)
Issaquah, WA 98027
206-392-8357
and:
N.E.E.D.S.
527 Charles Ave. 12A (APD)
Syracuse, NY 13209
800-634-1380
Fax 800-295-NEED (6333)

Cem Bond Paint

Odor-free; coats and seals concrete and masonry surfaces and exterior or interior wood trim
Available from:
AFM Enterprises, Inc.
1960 Chicago E7 (APD)
Riverside, CA 92507
909-781-6860
909-781-6861
Fax 909-781-6892
and:
Allergy Relief Shop,™Inc.
3371 Whittle Springs Rd. (APD)
Knoxville, TN 37917
Orders 800-626-2810
Questions 615-522-2795
and:
Allergy Resources
Mail: PO Box 888 (APD)
UPS: 264 Brookridge Ave. (APD)
Palmer Lake, CO 80133
Orders 800-USE-FLAX (873-3529)
Company plans a move; use 800 #

Asthma Resources Directory

Household Maintenance

and:
Flowright Int'l Products
1495 N.W. Gilman Blvd. #4 (APD)
Issaquah, WA 98027
206-392-8357

Drain Gun
Compressed air pump clears clogged drains without chemicals; sinks, toilets, bathtubs
Available from:
Brookstone Co.
5 Vose Farm Road (APD)
Peterborough, NH 03458
800-926-7000
Fax 603-924-0093

Dura Stain
Interior and exterior protective coating; shades of oak, maple, mahogany, walnut, birch, redwood, cedar, and clear
Available from:
AFM Enterprises, Inc.
1960 Chicago E7 (APD)
Riverside, CA 92507
909-781-6860
909-781-6861
Fax 909-781-6892
and:
Allergy Relief Shop,™Inc.
3371 Whittle Springs Rd. (APD)
Knoxville, TN 37917
Orders 800-626-2810
Questions 615-522-2795
and:
Flowright Int'l Products
1495 N.W. Gilman Blvd. #4 (APD)
Issaquah, WA 98027
206-392-8357
and:
N.E.E.D.S.
527 Charles Ave. 12A (APD)
Syracuse, NY 13209
800-634-1380
Fax 800-295-NEED (6333)

Dyno Flex Caulking Compound
Use as putty for windows, cracks, and repairs; can be applied over

asphalt shingles, roll roofing; repair seams and leaks on metal roofs and heating and air ducts
Available from:
AFM Enterprises, Inc.
1960 Chicago E7 (APD)
Riverside, CA 92507
909-781-6860
909-781-6861
Fax 909-781-6892
and:
Allergy Relief Shop,™Inc.
3371 Whittle Springs Rd. (APD)
Knoxville, TN 37917
Orders 800-626-2810
Questions 615-522-2795
and:
Flowright Int'l Products
1495 N.W. Gilman Blvd. #4 (APD)
Issaquah, WA 98027
206-392-8357

Dyno Flex
Water emulsion synthetic polymer system for use as a sealant and mastic compound; seals and repairs seams and leaks on metal roofs; natural, gray, and white
Available from:
AFM Enterprises, Inc.
1960 Chicago E7 (APD)
Riverside, CA 92507
909-781-6860
909-781-6861
Fax 909-781-6892
and:
Allergy Relief Shop,™Inc.
3371 Whittle Springs Rd. (APD)
Knoxville, TN 37917
Orders 800-626-2810
Questions 615-522-2795
and:
N.E.E.D.S.
527 Charles Ave. 12A (APD)
Syracuse, NY 13209
800-634-1380
Fax 800-295-NEED (6333)

Asthma Resources Directory
Household Maintenance

Dyno Seal

A liquid copolymer for use as a sealer and waterproof membrane; can be used below grade, under shower stalls and tubs, to repair or coat roofs; adheres to concrete, block, metal, wood, or asphalt shingles
Available from:
AFM Enterprises, Inc.
1960 Chicago E7 (APD)
Riverside, CA 92507
909-781-6860
909-781-6861
Fax 909-781-6892
and:
Allergy Relief Shop,™ Inc.
3371 Whittle Springs Rd. (APD)
Knoxville, TN 37917
Orders 800-626-2810
Questions 615-522-2795
and:
Flowright Int'l Products
1495 N.W. Gilman Blvd. #4 (APD)
Issaquah, WA 98027
206-392-8357
and:
N.E.E.D.S.
527 Charles Ave. 12A (APD)
Syracuse, NY 13209
800-634-1380
Fax 800-295-NEED (6333)

GT1000 Flat Latex Wall Paint

Formulated without slow releasing compounds or airborne fungicide; when dry, the preservative does not become airborne or leach out of the paint; low odor; "hypo-allergenic"; 9 stock colors, light tint bases
Available from:
Murco Wall Products, Inc.
300 N.E. 21st St. (APD)
Ft. Worth, TX 76106-8528
817-626-1987

Hard Seal

Odor-free, medium gloss sealer applies over previously painted surfaces to seal fumes and as finish coat on floors and cabinets

Available from:
AFM Enterprises, Inc.
1960 Chicago E7 (APD)
Riverside, CA 92507
909-781-6860
909-781-6861
Fax 909-781-6892
and:
Allergy Relief Shop,™ Inc.
3371 Whittle Springs Rd. (APD)
Knoxville, TN 37917
Orders 800-626-2810
Questions 615-522-2795
and:
Allergy Resources
Mail: PO Box 888 (APD)
UPS: 264 Brookridge Ave. (APD)
Palmer Lake, CO 80133
Orders 800-USE-FLAX (873-3529)
Company plans a move; use 800 #
and:
Flowright Int'l Products
1495 N.W. Gilman Blvd. #4 (APD)
Issaquah, WA 98027
206-392-8357
and:
N.E.E.D.S.
527 Charles Ave. 12A (APD)
Syracuse, NY 13209
800-634-1380
Fax 800-295-NEED (6333)

Interior Flat Latex 6450

Low odor; low biocide, produced without adding additional biocides during manufacture; free of fungicide and solvent; use on drywall, concrete, cement block, or primed wood; 8% gloss
Available from:
Miller Paint Co.
317 S.E. Grand Ave. (APD)
Portland, OR 97214
503-233-4021
Fax 503-238-6289

Interior Satin Latex 1450

Low odor; low biocide, produced without adding additional biocides during manufacture; free of fungicide

61

Asthma Resources Directory
Household Maintenance

and solvent; walls and ceilings; 15% gloss
Available from:
Miller Paint Co.
317 S.E. Grand Ave. (APD)
Portland, OR 97214
503-233-4021
Fax 503-238-6289

Interior Semi-Gloss Latex 2850
Low odor; low biocide, produced without adding additional biocides during manufacture; free of fungicide and solvent; walls and trim; kitchens, bathrooms; 50% gloss
Available from:
Miller Paint Co.
317 S.E. Grand Ave. (APD)
Portland, OR 97214
503-233-4021
Fax 503-238-6289

Joint Compound
Low odor joint and patching compound, low shrinkage; asbestos-free, fiber-free
Available from:
AFM Enterprises, Inc.
1960 Chicago E7 (APD)
Riverside, CA 92507
909-781-6860
909-781-6861
Fax 909-781-6892
and:
Allergy Relief Shop,™ Inc.
3371 Whittle Springs Rd. (APD)
Knoxville, TN 37917
Orders 800-626-2810
Questions 615-522-2795
and:
Flowright Int'l Products
1495 N.W. Gilman Blvd. #4 (APD)
Issaquah, WA 98027
206-392-8357
and:
N.E.E.D.S.
527 Charles Ave. 12A (APD)
Syracuse, NY 13209
800-634-1380
Fax 800-295-NEED (6333)

Klear Seal
Interior/exterior metal, masonry, and concrete sealer; glossy finish
Available from:
Flowright Int'l Products
1495 N.W. Gilman Blvd. #4 (APD)
Issaquah, WA 98027
206-392-8357
and:
N.E.E.D.S.
527 Charles Ave. 12A (APD)
Syracuse, NY 13209
800-634-1380
Fax 800-295-NEED (6333)

LE1000 High Gloss Latex Enamel
For kitchen, bathroom, woodwork; free of fungicide; low odor; "hypo-allergenic"; 9 stock colors, light tint bases
Available from:
Murco Wall Products, Inc.
300 N.E. 21st St. (APD)
Ft. Worth, TX 76106-8528
817-626-1987

Lift Off
Paint stripper; can be neutralized with water; removes paint, polymers, wax, asphalt, PVC plastics, fiber glass, adhesives, resins
Available from:
AFM Enterprises, Inc.
1960 Chicago E7 (APD)
Riverside, CA 92507
909-781-6860
909-781-6861
Fax 909-781-6892
and:
Allergy Relief Shop,™ Inc.
3371 Whittle Springs Rd. (APD)
Knoxville, TN 37917
Orders 800-626-2810
Questions 615-522-2795
and:
N.E.E.D.S.
527 Charles Ave. 12A (APD)
Syracuse, NY 13209
800-634-1380
Fax 800-295-NEED (6333)

Asthma Resources Directory
Household Maintenance

M-100 Hypo Joint Compound
Powdered, joint cement and texture compound; inert fillers, natural binders; free of preservatives, slow releasing compounds, asbestos; low odor; "hypo-allergenic"
Available from:
Murco Wall Products, Inc.
300 N.E. 21st St. (APD)
Ft. Worth, TX 76106-8528
817-626-1987

One Step Seal & Shine
Industrial/domestic sealer-polish; dries clear
Available from:
Flowright Int'l Products
1495 N.W. Gilman Blvd. #4 (APD)
Issaquah, WA 98027
206-392-8357
and:
N.E.E.D.S.
527 Charles Ave. 12A (APD)
Syracuse, NY 13209
800-634-1380
Fax 800-295-NEED (6333)

Paver Seal .003
Seals porous tile, conrete, and grout; helps control efflorescence
Available from:
AFM Enterprises, Inc.
1960 Chicago E7 (APD)
Riverside, CA 92507
909-781-6860
909-781-6861
Fax 909-781-6892
and:
Allergy Relief Shop,™ Inc.
3371 Whittle Springs Rd. (APD)
Knoxville, TN 37917
Orders 800-626-2810
Questions 615-522-2795
and:
N.E.E.D.S.
527 Charles Ave. 12A (APD)
Syracuse, NY 13209
800-634-1380
Fax 800-295-NEED (6333)

Penetrating Water Seal
Odor-free; reduces water absorption; helps control efflorescence; for porous bricks, some pavers, concrete, raw wood
Available from:
AFM Enterprises, Inc.
1960 Chicago E7 (APD)
Riverside, CA 92507
909-781-6860
909-781-6861
Fax 909-781-6892
and:
Allergy Relief Shop,™ Inc.
3371 Whittle Springs Rd. (APD)
Knoxville, TN 37917
Orders 800-626-2810
Questions 615-522-2795
and:
Allergy Resources
Mail: PO Box 888 (APD)
UPS: 264 Brookridge Ave. (APD)
Palmer Lake, CO 80133
Orders 800-USE-FLAX (873-3529)
Company plans a move; use 800 #
and:
Flowright Int'l Products
1495 N.W. Gilman Blvd. #4 (APD)
Issaquah, WA 98027
206-392-8357
and:
N.E.E.D.S.
527 Charles Ave. 12A (APD)
Syracuse, NY 13209
800-634-1380
Fax 800-295-NEED (6333)

Polyuraseal
Odor-free, clear gloss coating for floors, cabinets, and woodwork, metal, vinyl coated fabrics, plastic surfaces; substitute for polyurathane
Available from:
AFM Enterprises, Inc.
1960 Chicago E7 (APD)
Riverside, CA 92507
909-781-6860
909-781-6861
Fax 909-781-6892
and:

Asthma Resources Directory

Household Maintenance

Allergy Relief Shop,™Inc.
3371 Whittle Springs Rd. (APD)
Knoxville, TN 37917
Orders 800-626-2810
Questions 615-522-2795
and:
Allergy Resources
Mail: PO Box 888 (APD)
UPS: 264 Brookridge Ave. (APD)
Palmer Lake, CO 80133
Orders 800-USE-FLAX (873-3529)
Company plans a move; use 800 #
and:
Flowright Int'l Products
1495 N.W. Gilman Blvd. #4 (APD)
Issaquah, WA 98027
206-392-8357
and:
N.E.E.D.S.
527 Charles Ave. 12A (APD)
Syracuse, NY 13209
800-634-1380
Fax 800-295-NEED (6333)

Safecoat™ All Purpose Enamel

Water-base gloss enamel for interior and exterior walls, trim, woodwork, metal; water resisitant; white, bone
Available from:
AFM Enterprises, Inc.
1960 Chicago E7 (APD)
Riverside, CA 92507
909-781-6860
909-781-6861
Fax 909-781-6892
and:
Allergy Relief Shop,™Inc.
3371 Whittle Springs Rd. (APD)
Knoxville, TN 37917
Orders 800-626-2810
Questions 615-522-2795
and:
Flowright Int'l Products
1495 N.W. Gilman Blvd. #4 (APD)
Issaquah, WA 98027
206-392-8357
and:
N.E.E.D.S.
527 Charles Ave. 12A (APD)

Syracuse, NY 13209
800-634-1380
Fax 800-295-NEED (6333)

Safecoat™ Enamel

Odor-free, water-base semi-gloss enamel; bathroom, kitchen; white or bone, can be tinted
Available from:
AFM Enterprises, Inc.
1960 Chicago E7 (APD)
Riverside, CA 92507
909-781-6860
909-781-6861
Fax 909-781-6892
and:
Allergy Relief Shop,™Inc.
3371 Whittle Springs Rd. (APD)
Knoxville, TN 37917
Orders 800-626-2810
Questions 615-522-2795
and:
Allergy Resources
Mail: PO Box 888 (APD)
UPS: 264 Brookridge Ave. (APD)
Palmer Lake, CO 80133
Orders 800-USE-FLAX (873-3529)
Company plans a move; use 800 #
and:
Flowright Int'l Products
1495 N.W. Gilman Blvd. #4 (APD)
Issaquah, WA 98027
206-392-8357
and:
N.E.E.D.S.
527 Charles Ave. 12A (APD)
Syracuse, NY 13209
800-634-1380
Fax 800-295-NEED (6333)

Safecoat™ Paint

Low odor, non-reactive sealant and flat finish coat for walls and woodwork. Water base copolymer emulsion, odor-free; white, bone, and eight pastel colors; white can be tinted locally with Universal Tinting System.
Available from:
AFM Enterprises, Inc.
1960 Chicago E7 (APD)

Asthma Resources Directory
Household Maintenance

Riverside, CA 92507
909-781-6860
909-781-6861
Fax 909-781-6892
and:
Allergy Relief Shop,™ Inc.
3371 Whittle Springs Rd. (APD)
Knoxville, TN 37917
Orders 800-626-2810
Questions 615-522-2795
and:
Flowright Int'l Products
1495 N.W. Gilman Blvd. #4 (APD)
Issaquah, WA 98027
206-392-8357
and:
N.E.E.D.S.
527 Charles Ave. 12A (APD)
Syracuse, NY 13209
800-634-1380
Fax 800-295-NEED (6333)

Safecoat™ Primer
Odor-free, water-base primer for
walls, woodwork
Available from:
Allergy Resources
Mail: PO Box 888 (APD)
UPS: 264 Brookridge Ave. (APD)
Palmer Lake, CO 80133
Orders 800-USE-FLAX (873-3529)
Company plans a move; use 800 #
and:
AFM Enterprises, Inc.
1960 Chicago E7 (APD)
Riverside, CA 92507
909-781-6860
909-781-6861
Fax 909-781-6892
and:
Allergy Relief Shop,™ Inc.
3371 Whittle Springs Rd. (APD)
Knoxville, TN 37917
Orders 800-626-2810
Questions 615-522-2795
and:
Allergy Resources
Mail: PO Box 888 (APD)
UPS: 264 Brookridge Ave. (APD)
Palmer Lake, CO 80133

Orders 800-USE-FLAX (873-3529)
Company plans a move; use 800 #
and:
Flowright Int'l Products
1495 N.W. Gilman Blvd. #4 (APD)
Issaquah, WA 98027
206-392-8357
and:
N.E.E.D.S.
527 Charles Ave. 12A (APD)
Syracuse, NY 13209
800-634-1380
Fax 800-295-NEED (6333)

Sanding Sealer
Helps prevent bleed through of
oils, turpentines, and resins and
raising grain on wood when water-base
products are applied
Available from:
AFM Enterprises, Inc.
1960 Chicago E7 (APD)
Riverside, CA 92507
909-781-6860
909-781-6861
Fax 909-781-6892
and:
Allergy Relief Shop,™ Inc.
3371 Whittle Springs Rd. (APD)
Knoxville, TN 37917
Orders 800-626-2810
Questions 615-522-2795
and:
N.E.E.D.S.
527 Charles Ave. 12A (APD)
Syracuse, NY 13209
800-634-1380
Fax 800-295-NEED (6333)

Tile Grout
Substitute for cement-type
compounds; narrow joints on counter
tops and bath areas
Available from:
Flowright Int'l Products
1495 N.W. Gilman Blvd. #4 (APD)
Issaquah, WA 98027
206-392-8357

65

Asthma Resources Directory
Household Maintenance

Vinyl Block
Controls out-gassing from vinyl coverings in automobiles; liquid applies to any surface
Available from:
Flowright Int'l Products
1495 N.W. Gilman Blvd. #4 (APD)
Issaquah, WA 98027
206-392-8357

Wallpaper Adhesive
Use with wallpaper and vinyl wall covers
Available from:
Flowright Int'l Products
1495 N.W. Gilman Blvd. #4 (APD)
Issaquah, WA 98027
206-392-8357

Water Base Mexe Seal
Protects pavers from stain; applies to saltillo pavers, adobe, adoquin, grout, granite, concrete quarry tile, fired and unfired porcelain
Available from:
AFM Enterprises, Inc.
1960 Chicago E7 (APD)
Riverside, CA 92507
909-781-6860
909-781-6861
Fax 909-781-6892
and:
Allergy Relief Shop,™ Inc.
3371 Whittle Springs Rd. (APD)
Knoxville, TN 37917
Orders 800-626-2810
Questions 615-522-2795

and:
N.E.E.D.S.
527 Charles Ave. 12A (APD)
Syracuse, NY 13209
800-634-1380
Fax 800-295-NEED (6333)

Water Seal
Seals grout, tile, and concrete; coats porous surfaces, bare wood, painted surfaces, drywall, paneling, cabinets
Available from:
AFM Enterprises, Inc.
1960 Chicago E7 (APD)
Riverside, CA 92507
909-781-6860
909-781-6861
Fax 909-781-6892
and:
Allergy Relief Shop,™ Inc.
3371 Whittle Springs Rd. (APD)
Knoxville, TN 37917
Orders 800-626-2810
Questions 615-522-2795
and:
Flowright Int'l Products
1495 N.W. Gilman Blvd. #4 (APD)
Issaquah, WA 98027
206-392-8357
and:
N.E.E.D.S.
527 Charles Ave. 12A (APD)
Syracuse, NY 13209
800-634-1380
Fax 800-295-NEED (6333)

Allergy Products Directory

Copyrighted. Reproduction Prohibited by Law. 1259 El Camino #254, Menlo Park, CA 94025

Asthma Resources Directory
Irritant-free Pest Control

IRRITANT-FREE PEST CONTROL

PLANT PESTS IN THE GARDEN
PHYSICAL BARRIERS

Physical barriers can work well. Vegetable gum-based sticky barriers come in tubes. If you squeeze them on the ground around the trunk of bushes or trees, they can prevent garden ants from climbing up to tend aphids. When sticky barriers are squeezed around bedding plants, they can prevent snails and beetles from climbing up. These barriers are also available as sprays. Be sure they are vegetable-based.

Vegetable-based sticky barriers squeezed around bedding plants can keep snails and beetles away.

You will need to renew the barriers periodically. Try not to step in these gums and wear protective gloves because they are very sticky. For the same reason, keep children and pets away from these barriers.

If you put a barrier on the ground around the trunk of a tree that has a stake holding up the trunk, the ants will climb up the stake, transfer to the tree branches and tend the aphids. Squeeze the barrier around or on the stake as well.

Copper bands around the trunks of shrubs and trees also block snails. Surround a clump of plants with a raised border; generally, snails cannot climb over this barrier.

Remove the top and bottom of a used tin can and place the can over a seedling to protect it from cutworms and snails.

WASHING PLANTS

Directing a strong stream of water over plants to wash the leaves lowers somewhat populations of aphids, mealybugs, and spider mites. Do this early in the day and if you do it early in the season, you may keep the populations lower because all those removed insects would be unable to reproduce.

Washing also raises the humidity somewhat in the area and insects like spider mites prefer dusty, dirty plants and low humidity. Try weekly washings.

67

Asthma Resources Directory
Irritant-free Pest Control

SUGGESTIONS FOR PLANT PESTS

The following possible solutions have been gathered over the years from varying sources; you will find some more effective than others and many of them probably ineffective. We haven't tested these approaches and so cannot vouch for any of them.

- Weed Killer: 3- or 4-inch layer of mulch or several layers of newspaper, held down with stone, dirt or leaves

- Dandelions: baking soda and water or salt and water

- Weeds: hand weeding is the safest and most effective; be sure to remove the entire root system

- Weeds and Insects: in the fall, turn the soil over so that you expose wintering seeds and insect eggs and larvae to the drying air

- Slugs: beer in shallow dishes or newspaper rolls placed among plants that snails are damaging

- Snails: ginger or beer in shallow dishes or newspaper rolls placed among plants that snails are damaging

- Oil Spray for over-wintering insects: combine 1 cup cooking oil with 1 tablespoon liquid dish washing detergent or 1 1/2 teaspoons in 1 cup of water for aphids, beet armyworms, spider mites, and whiteflies. Do not use on cauliflower, red cabbage, or squash.

OUTDOOR PESTS

The most important part of controlling pests without irritating chemicals is to be sure that your environment is not attracting them. Garbage should be wrapped in air tight containers. Glass, metal, and paper should be rinsed

---
Be sure your environment is not attracting pests!
---

before disposal. Garbage cans should have tightly fitting lids. Garbage cans should not have holes in them and should be placed or fenced so that they cannot be moved or broken into by pets or other animals.

FLIES

Remember that traps attract flies to an area. Place your traps where flies are already a problem: near garbage, near pet areas, or in a far corner of your lot.

Asthma Resources Directory
Irritant-free Pest Control

There are several kinds of fly traps:

✔ Dehydrator traps simply keep flies imprisoned until they die.

✔ Jar traps, baited with raw meat for blow flies, have deflectors to prevent flies from escaping.

✔ Larger jar traps can be baited with a water-soluble pheromone (an attractant); you need to be sure you do not find this solution irritating.

✔ Traps with ultraviolet lights attract flies to electrically charged wire; these must be used in outbuildings like stables, barns, or kennels or in covered porches because flies cannot see ultraviolet in daylight.

There are many baits that seem to be attractive to flies. You want to be sure that you can tolerate them before using them. Also, most baits need to be moist in order to be effective. Try beer, beer with molasses, or ammonium carbonate and yeast for blow flies and stable flies

YELLOW JACKETS

Ground-nesting yellow jackets become problems if you are enjoying a barbecue, a picnic, are camping or swimming in a pool. They are attracted by food protein (barbecued food, drinks, and pet food) from about the time they become active as the weather warms until August. At that time, the population has grown considerably and sugar seems to attract them more: fruit trees, sodas, and juices.

Look for wasps inside a glass before drinking.

Move away from wasps if they are in the area. They will sting if you frighten them. Be careful when picking up a drink in a cup or glass without a lid; look inside to be sure no wasp is there.

Cleanliness is a good approach to making your home or camping area less attractive.

✔ Don't leave food or drinks uncovered outdoors.

✔ Rinse your food containers, papers, and packages before throwing them away.

✔ Garbage cans should not have holes in them; lids should be secure and fit tightly.

Place wasp traps downwind from seating areas.

Asthma Resources Directory
Irritant-free Pest Control

If you have cats and dogs, feed them indoors.

Although there are aerosol sprays designed to destroy wasps in their nests, the spray may be irritating and even if you are not sensitive to stings, you should probably have the nest handled by a professional.

Place traps downwind from where you will be eating outdoors. There are chemical and synthetic baits, but if you want to avoid possible irritation, you can use bologna, chicken, or pet food; in August use overripe fruit, jams, or sodas.

Send $1 to Bio-Integral Resource Center, PO Box 7414, (ARD) Berkeley 94707. Ask for their list of publications on safe controls of yellow jackets and other insects.

FOR FURTHER INFORMATION. . .

Natural Pest Control
Bruce Chapman, David Penman, and Phillip Hicks
Nelson Publications, Port Chester, NY

The Garden Pest Book
Bruce Chapman, David Penman, and Phillip Hicks
Nelson Publications, Port Chester, NY

Pests, Predators, and Pesticides
Jeanette Conacher
Available from Organic Growers' Association of Washington
Wembley, WA

Common Sense Pest Control Quarterly
Bio-Integral Resource Center, Berkeley, CA

Pests of Lanscape Trees and Shrubs
Univ. Of California, Agriculture/Natural Resources
Oakland, CA

Pests of the Garden and Small Farm: A Grower's Guide to Using Less Pesticide
Univ. Of California, Agriculture/Natural Resources
Oakland, CA

Natural Enemies Are Your Allies
Univ. Of California, Agriculture/Natural Resources
Oakland, CA

Biological Control in the Western United States
Univ. Of California, Agriculture/Natural Resources
Oakland, CA

INDOOR ENVIRONMENT

PETS

Many doctors who work with allergic and asthmatic patients recommend giving dogs and cats away, or at least letting them go on vacation while families see how their asthma or allergy symptoms respond to the absence of their pet.

Since it may take several months for your home to clear of pet allergens, most families decide too early that their pet is not causing any problem. Another difficulty is that other changes should be made to your home environment as well before symptom changes would be noted.

Pet saliva, dander, and urine are allergens.

Your pet's saliva can be a major cause of problems. If you are very sensitive, your skin may turn red and itch where your pet licks you, and cat saliva on fur aerosolizes and is found in the air.

Pet dander is another allergic problem. Although your pet's dander or skin flakes are an allergic component of house dust, they are also an allergen by themselves. Dander is a long-lasting problem. It can remain in a home that has not had a pet for months, even years.

FLEAS

If your doctor agrees that your pet can stay, you may still have problems from your pet's fleas.

Entomologist Ricahrd J. Brenner of the Agriculture Department's Medical and veterinary Entomology Research Lab in Gainesville, FL identified two flea-related proteins that can elicit allergic responses. Both come from flea debris: feces, eggshells, molted skin, and body parts. The researchers harvested these allergens from house dust vacuumed from the bedding, furniture, and carpeting of homes with fleas.

Many people are allergic to the proteins in the saliva of fleas and that's why a flea bite can trigger a runny nose and watery eyes.

SUGGESTONS FOR FLEAS

The SPCA recommends non toxic flea repellents for dogs made from herbal distillates. SPCA says they can also repel mosquitoes. These repellents are available in health food stores. Be careful because these herbs have odors of their

Asthma Resources Directory

Irritant-free Pest Control

own and can be irritating, so you may not be able to use them. If you have an allergy to spices, you also may not be

---

Herbs have odors of their own and can be irritating.

Some people have allergies to spices.

---

able to use them. These potential repellents include citronella, cedar wood, eucalyptus, pennyroyal, peppermint, orange, sassafras, lavender, geranium, clove, rue, mint. The oil is applied to your dog's fur or collar or added in small quantities to its regular shampoo. Don't use too much or your pet will end up with a dermatitis.

You can dust your dog with powdered sage, wormwood, sassafras, bay leaf, or vetiver. Wear a mask and gloves to try to prevent these powders from irritating your lungs or your skin. Remember, it is possible that these can also irritate you.

Nothing takes the place of regular washing of your pet's bedding and frequent vacuuming. Spraying sleeping areas and areas where your pet spends a lot of time like the car or the yard is usually recommended, but you should use caution and common sense before considering use of a spray and discuss such a move with your doctor.

Nothing takes the place of regular washing of your pet's bedding and frequent vacuuming.

We've been reading more and more that washing your cat either once a week in distilled water or twice a month in warm water or once a month in warm tap water or once a week in a special solution will stop or diminish your cat's production of skin protein.

Our first thought is exactly how are you going to set up a routine of washing your cat? Remember that your cat's saliva is a problem that isn't solved by a washing routine, and pet urine is another identified allergen.

INDOOR PESTS

Select your pest-control solution with care because of your own and your family's sensitivities, especially if you have young children or pets. Keep countertops and floor clean. Ants are attracted by grease and sugar; cockroaches and flies by food crumbs.

The following possible solutions have been gathered over the years from varying sources; you will find some more effective than others and many of them probably ineffective.

Asthma Resources Directory
Irritant-free Pest Control

We haven't tested these approaches and so cannot vouch for any of them.

Most importantly, your choice should depend upon your own sensitivities.

✔ Ants: mixtures of sugar with Epsom salts or sugar and boric acid or mint or spearmint or whole cloves or talcum powder or chalk lines or damp coffee grounds or salt and pepper or red chili pepper or paprika or borax or white rice and salt or honey and boric acid

✔ Beetles: store grains with a bay leaf or store them in the refrigerator in an airtight container

✔ Cockroaches: baking soda and powdered sugar or a mixture of flour, coca powder, and borax or cucumber rinds or bay leaves or a mixture of oatmeal and plaster of Paris or Epson salts with boric acid or plain baking soda or boric acid sprinkled along baseboards or oil of peppermint or eucalyptus or a mixture of flour, borax, cocoa and plaster of Paris

---

Most importantly, your choice of pest control should depend upon your own sensitivities.

✔ Fleas: Brewer's yeast added to pet food or salt in crevices of the dog house or sleeping area

✔ Flies: fly swatter or flypaper made from brown paper coated with a boiled mixture of corn syrup, sugar, and water or window and door screens or orange peels (no citrus allergy is present) or beer or beer with molasses or ammonium carbonate and yeast or fruit

✔ Moths: store clothes (clean and stain-free) in containers sealed with tape to make them airtight or lavender or whole peppercorns or Epsom salts or wrap in paper, freeze for one week and then store in tightly fitting bags or newspapers

✔ Rodents: clean counters and floors and seal holes; mousetraps or mixture of plaster of Paris, cocoa, powder and flour or garlic

✔ Silverfish: boric acid mixed with flour, sugar, and placed on strips of paper

HELP US TO HELP YOU

When writing to the companies and organizations listed here, tell them you saw them listed in *Allergy Products Directory.*

Asthma Resources Directory

Insect, Rodent Repellents

INSECT AND RODENT REPELLENTS

Pest control has been a problem over the centuries. This chapter presents possible methods of control that may be less likely to irritate lungs and skin. As always, what works for someone else may not work for you and what does not irritate you may not irritate pests either.

Catalogue companies may rotate their stock seasonally. If you see product here that is not in the current catalogue it may become available again during a more appropriate time of year for its use. You can always call the company to request the product. Catalogues generally like to stock for demand or they may be able to give you the name of the supplier.

Do not use hanging pest strips. They supply a constant release of pesticide into your air.

Electronic Flea Trap
Special light projecting onto a sticky surface lures adult fleas; attracts fleas from carpeting, not from pets; UL listed
Available from:
Home Trends
1450 Lyell Ave. (APD)
Rochester, NY 14606-2184
716-254-6520
Fax 716-458-9245

Gopher, Mole Eliminator
Aluminum stake vibrates, repels tunneling rodents (moles, gophers, voles); batteries
Available from:
Brookstone Co.
5 Vose Farm Road (APD)
Peterborough, NH 03458
800-926-7000
Fax 603-924-0093
and:
Home Trends
1450 Lyell Ave. (APD)
Rochester, NY 14606-2184
716-254-6520
Fax 716-458-9245

Insect Disposal System
Rechargeable vacuum-powered, hand-held tube sucks insects into nozzle and sealed, disposable cartridge; includes recharger; household current; on/off switch; unit made of ABS plastic
Available from:
Hammacher Schlemmer
147 E. 57th St. (APD)
New York, NY 10022
800-543-3366
212-421-9000
and:
Home Trends
1450 Lyell Ave. (APD)
Rochester, NY 14606-2184
716-254-6520
Fax 716-458-9245

Insect Eliminator
Fan-forced suction trap for mosquitoes, flies, moths, flying nsects; attractant ultraviolet light; water-filled retention tray; effective up to 1/2 acre; indoors, outdoors; household current
Available from:
Hammacher Schlemmer
147 E. 57th St. (APD)
New York, NY 10022
800-543-3366
212-421-9000

Insectigone®
Odor-free diatomaceous earth
Available from:
Home Trends

Asthma Resources Directory
Insect, Rodent Repellents

1450 Lyell Ave. (APD)
Rochester, NY 14606-2184
716-254-6520
Fax 716-458-9245

Mosquito Hawk

Imitates sound of a dragonfly's wings; range of 50 ft.; 9 volt battery
Available from:
Lifestyle Fascination
55 Progress Pl. (APD)
Jackson, NJ 08527-3002
800-669-0987
908-928-1800
Fax 908-928-1107

Over Nite® Flea Trap

Automatic, photo cell-operated night light draws fleas to a disposble, sticky surface; UL listed; does not remove fleas from pets
Available from:
Home Trends
1450 Lyell Ave. (APD)
Rochester, NY 14606-2184
716-254-6520
Fax 716-458-9245

Pest Trap

Box with a natural lure attracts insects that infest grains, flours, nuts, pet foods; sticky surface traps insects; for use in cabinets
Available from:
Vermont Country Store,® The
PO Box 3000 (APD)
Manchester Center, VT 05255-3000
802-362-2400
Fax 802-362-0285

PestChaser

High frequency tones repel rodents and insects; internal transformer; household current; UL listed
Available from:
Home Trends
1450 Lyell Ave. (APD)
Rochester, NY 14606-2184
716-254-6520

Fax 716-458-9245
and:
Plow & Hearth
301 Madison Rd. (APD)
PO Box 830 (APD)
Orange, VA 22960
800-627-1712
Fax 800-843-2509

PestContro™

Uses magnetic pulses and sonic waves; for ants, spiders, roaches, mice, rats; plugs into electric outlet
Available from:
Lifestyle Fascination
55 Progress Pl. (APD)
Jackson, NJ 08527-3002
800-669-0987
908-928-1800
Fax 908-928-1107

Protector, The™

Electronic pulse kills flies, other flying insects; FDA-permitted use in food preparation areas; emits attractant light with wavelength and flicker detected by insects; disposble adhesive pad trap; indoors
Available from:
Frontgate
4850 Smith Rd. (APD)
PO Box 0613 (APD)
Cincinnati, OH 45264-0613
800-626-6488
Fax 800-436-2105

Stainless Steel Bug Light

Black lights attract insects, house flies; electric charge protected by safety shield; protects 1-1/2 acres; 11-3/8"x11-3/8"x30;" 30 lbs.
Available from:
Sporty's® Preferred Living
Clermont County Airport (APD)
Batavia, OH 45103-9747
800-543-8633
Fax 513-732-6560

Asthma Resources Directory

Insect, Rodent Repellents

Stinger Laser
Attracts light-sensitive flying insects to electrically charged grid; UV 40; rust-proof; UL listed
Available from:
Stinger Environmental Products
Div. of Dejaz® Corp.
Rt. 3, Box 46 (APD)
Greeneville, TN 37743

SureFire Yellow Jacket Trap
Hang near gathering area, but away from people; bright yellow color and partially cooked piece of meat are attractants; to reuse, unfold bottom and empty
Available from:
Brookstone Co.
5 Vose Farm Road (APD)
Peterborough, NH 03458
800-926-7000
Fax 603-924-0093
and:
Solutions®
PO Box 6878 (APD)
Portland, OR 97228
800-342-9988
Fax 503-643-1973

Terra Fly Catchers
Composed of mineral oil and rubber; four ribbons per package
Available from:
Allergy Relief Shop,™ Inc.
3371 Whittle Springs Rd. (APD)
Knoxville, TN 37917
Orders 800-626-2810
Questions 615-522-2795

Terra Fly Swatters
Wire with cloth blade and wire handles
Available from:
Allergy Relief Shop,™ Inc.
3371 Whittle Springs Rd. (APD)
Knoxville, TN 37917
Orders 800-626-2810
Questions 615-522-2795

Transonic ESP
Electronic, ultrasonic emitter; covers up to 10,000 sq. ft.
Available from:
Lifestyle Fascination
55 Progress Pl. (APD)
Jackson, NJ 08527-3002
800-669-0987
908-928-1800
Fax 908-928-1107

Transonic® IXL Pest Repeller
High-intensity sound higher than human perception reaches to 2,000 sq. ft.; rats, mice, bats, moquitoes, spiders, fleas; household current
Available from:
Solutions®
PO Box 6878 (APD)
Portland, OR 97228
800-342-9988
Fax 503-643-1973

Ultrasonic Flea Collar
Ultrasonic sound repells fleas, ticks; nylon collar for cats (elastic to prevent choking), dogs; replaceable lithium battery
Available from:
Hammacher Schlemmer
147 E. 57th St. (APD)
New York, NY 10022
800-543-3366
212-421-9000

Wasp/Yellow Jacket Trap
Hang near gathering area, but away from people; odorless sugar water attracts and traps stinging wasps and yellow jackets
Available from:
Brookstone Co.
5 Vose Farm Road (APD)
Peterborough, NH 03458
800-926-7000
Fax 603-924-0093

Asthma Resources Directory

Insect, Rodent Repellents

Whitefly Traps

Vegetable-based, sticky film on yellow card attracts whiteflies and gnats
Available from:
Home Trends
1450 Lyell Ave. (APD)
Rochester, NY 14606-2184
716-254-6520
Fax 716-458-9245

Yard Gard

Ultrasonic waves repel unwanted animals; various frequencies cover area up to 80'x50'

Available from:
Home Trends
1450 Lyell Ave. (APD)
Rochester, NY 14606-2184
716-254-6520
Fax 716-458-9245
and:
Plow & Hearth
301 Madison Rd. (APD)
PO Box 830 (APD)
Orange, VA 22960
800-627-1712
Fax 800-843-2509

HELP US TO HELP YOU

When writing to the companies and organizations listed here, be sure to use the initials (APD) as part of the address and tell them you saw them listed in *Allergy Products Directory.*

If you call, be sure to tell them you found them in *Allergy Products Directory.*

This is important to you because:

1. Lets the company know that its listings have helped you.

2. Encourages the company to keep *Allergy Products Directory* informed of its new products so that we can keep you informed.

3. Enables us to keep our listings accurate and up-to-date for you on the latest products, services, and innovations.

4. Enables us to keep the Directory price low for you.

Thank you for your help.

77

Allergy Products Directory

Copyrighted. Reproduction Prohibited by Law. 1259 El Camino #254,Menlo Park, CA 94025

Asthma Resources Directory

Pulmonary Function

PULMONARY FUNCTION MEASUREMENTS

Your doctor wants to know how well your lungs do their job of moving air in and out. He or she will use a spirometer which measures and then evaluates your pulmonary function.

Breathing tests will tell your doctor if you have a problem, what kind of problem you have, and how much of a problem you have.

Your results are measured against people without problems who are your age, size, and weight. Your results are a percentage of their results.

PULMONARY FUNCTION TESTING

Asthma by definition is reversible lung disease. Therefore, lung volumes are measured before and after a medication that relaxes muscles around the airways and "opens" the airways.

If you have asthma, your test will show a decrease in the amount of air moving in and out of your lungs as well as a decrease in the speed with which it moves.

If you have asthma, your test will show a decrease in the amount of air moving in and out of your lungs as well as a decrease in the speed with which it moves. There are other measurements your doctor can make (which are explained below) and you can improve these measurements by inhaling a bronchodilator, a medication that relaxes your bronchial tubes.

SPIROMETERS

Pulmonary function tests are used by your doctor to diagnose asthma and measure lung volumes. You blow air from your mouth into a tube that is connected to a spirometer. The spirometer measures the amount of air that moves in and out of your lungs and how fast that air moves.

Spriometers measure the volulme that is exhaled from the lung; tidal volume, vital capacity, expiratory reserve, volume inspiratory capacity. One type of spirometer is a

Allergy Products Directory
Copyrighted. Reproduction Prohibited by Law. 1259 El Camino #254, Menlo Park, CA 94025

Asthma Resources Directory
Pulmonary Function

bell displaced by air over water. Another type uses a wedge or bellows.

Vital capacity is most important. To determine whether the reduction in vital capacity is due to restriction or obstruction, measurements of flow rate are obtained. Flow rates are measured directly or determined by noting the volume expired over a period of time. Timed volumes measured on the spirometer include PEFR. FVC FEV MMEF and are described below.

SPIROMETER MEASUREMENTS

TIDAL VOLUME:

How much air you breath in and out when you are relaxed and not paying attention

INSPIRATORY RESERVE:

After you have inhaled normally, how much more air can you inhale when you force yourself to inhale more and try as hard as you possibly can?

EXPIRATORY RESERVE:

After you have exhaled normally, how much more air can you exhale when you force yourself to exhale more and you try as hard as you possibly can?

VITAL CAPACITY:

The amount of air you are utilizing when you take the biggest possible breath that you can and then blow out forcibly for as hard and as long as you can

FORCED VITAL CAPACITY (FVC) or FORCED EXPIRATORY VOLUME:

This is a measurement of the maximum amount of air you can push out of your lungs with force and speed after inhaling as much as you possibly can.

FORCED EXPIRATORY VOLUME IN ONE SECOND (FEV1):

The amount of air forcefully exhaled in the first second after you have inhaled as much as you can.

Asthma Resources Directory

Pulmonary Function

PEAK EXPIRATORY FLOW RATE (PEFR):

How fast you can move the air out of your lungs when you exhale as fast as you can?

FORCED EXPIRATORY FLOW 25-75 (FEF 25-75):

This is a measurement of the mid-part of your air flow while you are forcing exhalation.

RESIDUAL VOLUME:

The amount of air that remains in your lungs after you forcibly blow out as much as you possibly can

BRONCHIAL PROVOCATION TEST

Another type of pulmonary function test is the bronchial provocation test. If you have asthma, this test can be used to measure the amount of airway obstruction or wheezing produced when you inhale a chemical mist the doctor gives you.

Your measurements will show a decrease in how fast the air moves out of your lungs and how much air you are able to exhale. You can then be given a bronchodilator to relax your lungs. This test is only done when lungs are "stable."

EXERCISE PROVOCATION MEASUREMENTS

A second type of provocation test is the measurement of lung volumes during and after exercise. This may be done in a doctor's office or at any exercise facility or at home. You can check your own peak flow during and after exercise and at home.

IMPORTANCE OF THE PEAK FLOW RATE

The National Heart, Lung, and Blood Institute guidelines for asthma call for prevention and prevention depends upon patient education, peak flow meter monitoring, and anti-inflammatory drugs.

With the early warning of your peak flow meter, you can start medication immediately to avoid an asthma attack.

When your airways start to close down, your flow rate reading will drop. If it drops 10%, you may be in the early stages of an asthma attack. Think of it as an early warning signal. When you are wheezing, you are already down 25 to 50%.

You should find your own "normal" peak flow and not rely on values based on height and sex. Dr. Thomas Plaut has written that he prefers "personal best peak flow" to "normal" peak flow. To find it, measure two days when your asthma is under control and use that measurement as your standard.

With the early warning of your peak flow meter, you can start medication immediately to avoid an attack. You can monitor your condition with peak flow readings. In conjunction with your Asthma Plan worked out with your doctor, your readings can help you decide to call your doctor or go to the emergency room.

The guidelines call for peak flow readings twice a day until asthma is in control and then daily or at least three times a week. Your doctor's office will explain the use of the peak flow meter to you. Be sure that you or your child understand how to use it.

Allergy Products Directory

Copyrighted. Reproduction Prohibited by Law. 1259 El Camino #254, Menlo Park, CA 94025

Asthma Resources Directory
Bronchodilator Medications

BRONCHODILATOR MEDICATIONS

Bronchodilators are frequently prescribed for asthma patients. They are usually considered safe when be used properly. You will generally need a doctor's prescription for your medication. Some inhalers with epinephrine are available over the counter, but do not use them unless your doctor specifically tells you to and you have been diagnosed with asthma. They cause more side effects than prescription medications, according to Joann Blessing-Moore, MD.

Bronchodilators are not a cure for asthma.

They can relieve symptoms by opening air passages in the lungs.

Bronchodilators are not a cure for asthma. They can relieve symptoms by opening air passages in the lungs to allow easier breathing, relieve wheezing, coughing, shortness of breath, and tightness in the chest. They can prevent bronchospasm when taken shortly before exercising. Symptom relief can be almost immediate — within a few seconds — or up to 30 minutes, for long-acting preparations.

The most common way to administer bronchodilators is with the metered-dose inhaler. A Freon-driven jet, sprays a controlled amount of medication through a mouthpiece which you inhale.

Your doctor will give you careful instructions as to the proper use of this inhaler. You should be sure that you and your child understand how to use the inhaler. Practice and demonstrate your technique to a doctor or nurse before leaving the office.

Always follow your doctor's instructions regarding how many puffs to take and how often to use the inhaler.

Dosage varies depending upon symptoms and other factors. Always follow your doctor's instructions regarding how many puffs to take and how often to use the inhaler.

Bronchodilators can also be taken by nebulizers to produce the spray.

If you miss a dose, take it as soon as you remember and ask your doctor about taking your next dose. You do not

Asthma Resources Directory
Bronchodilator Medications

want to take more of the medication than is recommended because serious side effects can result.

SIDE EFFECTS

Side effects include nervousness, restlessness, and trembling. Less common side effects are coughing, dizziness, indigestion, irritated mouth or throat, pounding heartbeat, headache, increased sweating, an increase in blood pressure, muscle cramps, twitching, nausea, vomiting, sleeplessness, pallor, and weakness. Contact your doctor if you develop these effects.

If the medication leaves an unpleasant taste in your mouth or you notice a change in your sense of smell or taste, talk to your doctor.

PRECAUTIONS

Tell your doctor if. . .

- Your bronchospasm continues
- You are pregnant. Ask about additional risks
- You will be breast-feeding. Ask about additional risks
- You are diabetic and notice a change in sugar test results
- You have had adverse reactions to any drugs or other adrenergic bronchodilators
- You have other medical problems such as heart disease, vascular disease, high blood pressure, overactive thyroid, Parkinson's disease
- You are taking any other prescription drugs, particularly beta blockers, heart medicines, or mood-changing drugs
- You are taking any over-the-counter drugs
- You have ever used stimulants, including cocaine

Allergy Products Directory
Copyrighted. Reproduction Prohibited by Law. 1259 El Camino #254, Menlo Park, CA 94025

Asthma Resources Directory
Respiratory Tools

RESPIRATORY TOOLS

Inhaling medications allows your medicine to go directly into your lungs (the location of your problem) and start helping you faster than if you were to take them by mouth. You also need less medication when you can inhale it and you will experience fewer side effects.

Be sure you are trained, observed, and coached to use your respiratory tool.

Be sure that you are trained in the use of your respiratory tool and that your technique is observed. You want to be sure that you are using your equipment properly and that you are getting the full benefit of your medication. Written instructions are not sufficient. Be sure someone observes you and coaches you.

METERED DOSE INHALERS

A metered dose inhaler is a cartridge filled with medication. It either propels a measured dose of your medicine out with an inactive gas carrier (Freon) or turns the dose into a spray by passing air over a solution of medication. Each puff of medication is exactly measured.

✔ Remove the cap.

✔ Shake your metered dose inhaler two or three times. Hold it with the cartridge vertical and higher than your mouth. Bring it close to your open mouth, but do not close your lips around the mouth piece.

✔ Exhale as completely as you can. Press down on the cartridge and start inhaling slowly until your lungs are filled. Hold your breath, count slowly to 10, then breathe out slowly. Repeat these steps for a second inhalation, if prescribed.

Try to keep your inhaler warm when you are outdoors in cold weather. The propellant gas inside the inhaler contracts when cold and may not be capable of providing you with your full dose of medication. If you are outdoors for extended periods, use a full inhaler and roll it between your hands to warm it.

Alternatively, try to take your medication before you go outside, or enter a warm building for several minutes to warm your canister. Be sure to shake the canister before using it.

Asthma Resources Directory

Respiratory Tools

If you have mild to moderate asthma, metered dose inhalers can give you mobility and freedom from the need to plug in your nebulizer to an electric outlet. You can hold your inhaler in your hand and carry it in a pocket.

The major problem with inhalers is that they require good inhalation technique. The reason that the spacer is so important is that the "jet" of medication out of the metered dose inhaler is powered very, very rapidly by Freon. Most of the medication hits the back of the throat, never reaching the lungs.

There are devices that will solve the problem of coordinating inhalation with medication delivery. These devices are nebulizers, dry powder inhalers, holding tubes, and spacers.

Nebulizers, dry powder inhalers, spacers, and holding tubes
Solve the problem of coordinating inhalation
with medication delivery.

SOLVING THE INHALATION AND DELIVERY PROBLEM
NEBULIZERS

Nebulizers produce a fine mist with your asthma medication. A compressor creates a mist by passing air through your medication so quickly and at such a high frequency that the particles produced are extremely small.

You put the mouth piece inside your mouth or put the mask on and take slow, deep breaths at your own pace while the nebulizer delivers its fine mist of medication continuously.

This approach works well for very young children, for adults who may have difficulty with metered dose inhalers, and with the elderly who may prefer to proceed at their own pace.

✔ Nebulizers can be purchased with:

✔ Carrying cases

✔ Car battery attachments

✔ And/or their own battery options (if electricity is unavailable or you live in an   area with frequent black-outs.

Keep your nebulizer clean so that it can give you the correct dosage of medication. Bacteria can grow on the mouth piece of dirty nebulizers. Disassemble the

Asthma Resources Directory

Respiratory Tools

equipment; soak it in a mild vinegar solution. Rinse and let air dry on a clean towel or cloth.

Keep your nebulizer clean so that it can give you the correct dosage of medication.

Bacteria can grow on the mouth piece of dirty nebulizers.

Follow your doctor's instructions for setting up your nebulizer, measuring your medication, filling it, using it, and cleaning it.

DRY POWDER INHALERS

This group of inhalers allows the user to pierce the container holding powdered medication first and then to inhale, thereby eliminating the need to coordinate medication delivery and inhalation.

SPACERS OR ADAPTERS

An adapter or spacer is a tube or collapsible bag that holds the medication between the inhaler and your mouth.

The spacer solves several problems: coordinating your inhalation with the compression of the inhaler and being sure that the medication ends up where it belongs in the bronchioles, rather than the back of your mouth.

On days when you are having difficulty breathing, the adapter makes it easier to inhale your medication. For these reasons, everyone using a metered dose inhaler should use an adapter.

To take your medication with a spacer, first puff the medication into the spacer and then inhale over three seconds. Hold your breath for ten seconds. Put one puff into the spacer at a time.

BUBBLE RESERVOIR

One type of spacer, the bubble reservoir, was specifically designed for children with mild to moderate asthma. The bubble holds the medication until your child is ready to breathe in.

Your child may take as many breaths as needed in order to inhale the entire amount of medication. The medication traveling into the air chamber loses much of its unpleasant taste.

86

The bubble reservoir also contains a float that is a visual indication that the medication is working. As the airways open with the inhalation of the medication, the child is able to inhale more deeply and the float moves higher.

TUBE RESERVOIR

A second type of spacer is the tube reservoir. The tube is about 8-inches long and 2-inches in diameter and holds the medicated mist until it is inhaled. A valve prevents accidental release of medication.

BREATH CONTROLLLED INHALER

Another method of avoiding the timing problem associated with metered dose inhalers is an inhaler that is breath actuated. That is, when you start to breathe in, the inhaler starts to deliver the medication.

FLICK ADAPTER

Compressing a hand-held inhaler can be a problem for those with arthritis or other muscular or nerve problems. This adapter can deliver the medicated puff with a flick of the finger.

PEAK FLOW METERS

A change in air flow may be detected before a change in pulmonary function. A peak flow meter measures these early changes in larger airway function, not the changes that can occur in the small branches of the lungs.

A peak flow meter measures your peak expiratory flow or how fast you can exhale air when you force yourself to exhale. You only need a hard, fast blow for a few seconds; this is not a pulmonary function test. Ideal rates vary depending upon your height and age. You can find yours by taking several readings when you are feeling fine.

Follow your doctor's instructions about taking readings and recording them. Readings taken in the morning and in the evening, before and after medications, and when feeling tightness of the chest will help you assess the effectiveness of your medications.

In general, peak flow measurements done in the morning will often be lower than in the evening. Peak flow

Asthma Resources Directory

Respiratory Tools

measurements should be higher after medications. The lungs are normally "at their best" at four pm and at the lowest lung volumes at four am. If there is asthma or bronchial obstruction, the four am drop becomes even more notable. If you or your child awake wheezing in the early morning hours, be sure to let your doctor know so that medication can be altered.

HOW TO USE YOUR PEAK FLOW METER

Guidelines for the Diagnosis and Management of Asthma: Technique for Measurement recommends readings in the morning and in the evening.

1. Set the indicator to the bottom of the scale or to zero.

2. Stand up.

3. Hold the meter parallel to the ground.

4. Take a deep breath.

5. Close your lips tightly around the mouthpiece.

6. Be sure your tongue does not block the opening of the meter.

7. Blow out as hard and as fast as you can.

8. The indicator now shows your peak flow. Write down that number.

9. Repeat two more times.

10. Enter the highest reading in your chart, including date and time.

Keep the meter clean. Use warm, soapy water; rinse completely and let dry. Store properly. If your meter has a spring and you use your meter frequently, you may need to replace the spring yearly.

Once you start keeping track of your peak flow rates, you can play detective.

You can see if a particular perfume or animal or smoke changes your peak expiratory flow rate.

You can check certain signs or feelings you experience to see if they are also early warning signs of a change in your peak flow rate.

You can also keep tabs on the effectiveness of your medication dosage. Does your measurement improve after therapy?

Asthma Resources Directory

Respiratory Tools

You and your doctor will devise a plan of action for you when your morning peak expiratory flow reading is low. Such a reading could indicate the start of an asthma attack or the start of a cold. You should keep the telephone number of your doctor with your records and an alternate number as well in case he or she is not on call. A more detailed plan is discussed in the chapter *Talking to Your Doctor.*

Peak flow zones used by many physicians are:

GREEN zone: Normal lung function

YELLOW zone 70-80% of normal. Add medications for stability

RED Zone: 50% of normal. Contact MD or go to emergency room

> **Use of a peak flow meter can help you decide when to add or when to subtract medications and when to seek help. It can also help determine how effective medications are.**

Allergy Products Directory
Copyrighted. Reproduction Prohibited by Law. 1259 El Camino #254, Menlo Park, CA 94025

Asthma Resources Directory

Respiratory Aids

RESIRATORY AIDS

PEAK FLOW METERS

Assess® Low Range/Pediatric Peak Flow Meter

HealthScan pediatric meter accurate to plus or minus 5%; 30 to 390 liters per minute; normal value tables; monitors on visual indicator with readable scale; recording chart; adult and pediatric disposable mouthpieces; polycarbonate plastic; dishwasher safe; carrying case
Available from:
Allergy Control Products, Inc.
96 Danbury Rd. (APD)
PO Box 793 (APD)
Ridgefield, CT 06877
800-422-DUST (3878)
203-438-9580
Fax 203-431-8963
and:
Allergy Supply Co., Inc. The
11994 Star Court (APD)
Herndon, VA 22071
800-323-6744
Metropolitan DC 703-391-2011
Fax 703-391-2014
BBS 703-521-0638
and:
American Allergy Supply
PO Box 722022 (APD)
Houston, TX 77272-2022
800-321-1096
713-995-6110
and:
American Allergy Supply
PO Box 722022 (APD)
Houston, TX 77272-2022
800-321-1096
713-995-6110
and:
HealthScan Products, Inc.
908 Pompton Ave. (APD)
Cedar Grove, NJ 07009-1292
800-962-1266
In NJ 201-857-3414
and:

National Allergy Supply, Inc.
4400 Georgia Hwy. 120 (APD)
PO Box 1658 (APD)
Duluth, GA 30136
800-522-1448
In Atlanta 404-623-8077
Fax 404-623-5568
and:
Vacumetrics
Vacu-Med
4483 McGrath St. #102 (APD)
Ventura, CA 93003
800-235-3333
805-644-7461
Fax 805-654-8759

Assess® Standard Peak Flow Meter

Available from:
Aller-Guard,® Inc.
Southgate Office Park
1645 S.W. 41st St. (APD)
Topeka, KS 66609-1250
800-234-0816
913-267-9333
Fax 913-267-0072
and:
Allergy Asthma Technology
4151 N. Kedzie (APD)
PO Box 18398 (APD)
Chicago, IL 60618
800-621-5545
312-465-8020
Fax 312-465-7619
and:
Allergy Clean Environments
501 Station Ave. (APD)
Haddon Heights, NJ 08035
800-882-4110
In NJ 609-546-1101
Fax 609-546-1466
URL:
http:\\WWW.infomall.com\allergy.html
and:
Allergy Control Products, Inc.
96 Danbury Rd. (APD)
PO Box 793 (APD)

Asthma Resources Directory

Respiratory Aids

Ridgefield, CT 06877
800-422-DUST (3878)
203-438-9580
Fax 203-431-8963
and:
Allergy Supply Co., Inc. The
11994 Star Court (APD)
Herndon, VA 22071
800-323-6744
Metropolitan DC 703-391-2011
Fax 703-391-2014
BBS 703-521-0638
and:
American Allergy Supply
PO Box 722022 (APD)
Houston, TX 77272-2022
800-321-1096
713-995-6110
and:
Environtrol® Corp.
PO Box 31313 (APD)
St. Louis, MO 63131
800-423-1982
In St. Louis 314-966-6886
and:
HealthScan Products, Inc.
908 Pompton Ave. (APD)
Cedar Grove, NJ 07009-1292
800-962-1266
In NJ 201-857-3414
and:
National Allergy Supply, Inc.
4400 Georgia Hwy. 120 (APD)
PO Box 1658 (APD)
Duluth, GA 30136
800-522-1448
In Atlanta 404-623-8077
Fax 404-623-5568
and:
Vacumetrics
Vacu-Med
4483 McGrath St. #102 (APD)
Ventura, CA 93003
800-235-3333
805-644-7461
Fax 805-654-8759

Astech™ Peak Flow Meter

Color coded, adjustable indicators, red, yellow, and green, show personalized safe and danger zones; adult and pediatric use; aluminum for durability
Available from:
Allergy & Asthma Network/
Mothers of Asthmatics, Inc.
3554 Chain Bridge Rd. Ste 200 (APD)
Fairfax, VA 22030-2709
Orders 800-878-4403
703-385-4403
Fax 703-352-4354
and:
Allergy Clean Environments
501 Station Ave. (APD)
Haddon Heights, NJ 08035
800-882-4110
In NJ 609-546-1101
Fax 609-546-1466
URL:
http:\\WWW.infomall.com\allergy.html
and:
Allergy Control Products, Inc.
96 Danbury Rd. (APD)
PO Box 793 (APD)
Ridgefield, CT 06877
800-422-DUST (3878)
203-438-9580
Fax 203-431-8963
and:
Center Laboratories
35 Channel Dr. (APD)
PO Box 70 (APD)
Port Washington, NY 11050
Customer service 800-223-6837

Asthma Alert Monitor

Preset monitor to individual's normal peak flow; monitor whistles when peak flow is achieved; scale from 1 to 10 liters per second 960-600 LPM; includes explanatory booklet, instruuctions for monitoring
Available from:
Vacumetrics
Vacu-Med
4483 McGrath St. #102 (APD)
Ventura, CA 93003

Asthma Resources Directory

Respiratory Aids

800-235-3333
805-644-7461
Fax 805-654-8759

mini-Wright® Low Range Peak Flow Meter PF-240

Clement-Clarke low range meter from 30 to 370 liters per minute; at home monitoring of Peak Expiratory Flow; adult and pediatric disposable, sterilizable mouthpieces with tapered design; portable, plastic carrying case; 11 oz.; daily record charts
Available from:
Allergy & Asthma Network/
Mothers of Asthmatics, Inc.
3554 Chain Bridge Rd. Ste 200 (APD)
Fairfax, VA 22030-2709
Orders 800-878-4403
703-385-4403
Fax 703-352-4354
and:
Allergy Asthma Technology
4151 N. Kedzie (APD)
PO Box 18398 (APD)
Chicago, IL 60618
800-621-5545
312-465-8020
Fax 312-465-7619
and:
Allergy Supply Co., Inc. The
11994 Star Court (APD)
Herndon, VA 22071
800-323-6744
Metropolitan DC 703-391-2011
Fax 703-391-2014
BBS 703-521-0638
and:
Armstrong Medical Industries, Inc.
375 Knightsbridge Pkwy. (APD)
PO Box 700 (APD)
Lincolnshire, IL 60069
800-323-4220
In IL 708-913-0101
Fax 708-913-0138
Western States 800-442-6991
Western States Fax 619-535-0525
and:
Armstrong Medical Industries, Inc.
375 Knightsbridge Pkwy. (APD)

PO Box 700 (APD)
Lincolnshire, IL 60069
800-323-4220
In IL 708-913-0101
Fax 708-913-0138
Western States 800-442-6991
Western States Fax 619-535-0525
and:
Clement Clark, Inc.
3128-D E. 17th Ave. (APD)
Columbus, OH 43219
800-848-8923
614-478-2777
Fax 614-478-2622
and:
Dura Pharmaceuticals, Inc.
PO Box 2209 (APD)
Ramona, CA 92065-0938
800-231-3195
In CA 619-789-6840
and:
National Allergy Supply, Inc.
4400 Georgia Hwy. 120 (APD)
PO Box 1658 (APD)
Duluth, GA 30136
800-522-1448
In Atlanta 404-623-8077
Fax 404-623-5568

mini-Wright® Peak Flow Meter PF-239

Clement Clarke regular range meter from 60 to 800 liters per minute; at home monitoring of Peak Expiratory Flow; adult and pediatric disposable, sterilizable mouthpieces with tapered design; portable, plastic carrying case; 11 oz.; daily record charts
Available from:
Allergy & Asthma Network/
Mothers of Asthmatics, Inc.
3554 Chain Bridge Rd. Ste 200 (APD)
Fairfax, VA 22030-2709
Orders 800-878-4403
703-385-4403
Fax 703-352-4354
and:
Allergy Asthma Technology
4151 N. Kedzie (APD)
PO Box 18398 (APD)

Asthma Resources Directory

Respiratory Aids

Chicago, IL 60618
800-621-5545
312-465-8020
Fax 312-465-7619
and:
Allergy Supply Co., Inc. The
11994 Star Court (APD)
Herndon, VA 22071
800-323-6744
Metropolitan DC 703-391-2011
Fax 703-391-2014
BBS 703-521-0638
and:
Armstrong Medical Industries, Inc.
375 Knightsbridge Pkwy. (APD)
PO Box 700 (APD)
Lincolnshire, IL 60069
800-323-4220
In IL 708-913-0101
Fax 708-913-0138
Western States 800-442-6991
Western States Fax 619-535-0525
and:
Clement Clark, Inc.
3128-D E. 17th Ave. (APD)
Columbus, OH 43219
800-848-8923
614-478-2777
Fax 614-478-2622
and:
Clement Clark, Inc.
3128-D E. 17th Ave. (APD)
Columbus, OH 43219
800-848-8923
614-478-2777
Fax 614-478-2622
and:
Dura Pharmaceuticals, Inc.
PO Box 2209 (APD)
Ramona, CA 92065-0938
800-231-3195
In CA 619-789-6840
and:
National Allergy Supply, Inc.
4400 Georgia Hwy. 120 (APD)
PO Box 1658 (APD)
Duluth, GA 30136
800-522-1448
In Atlanta 404-623-8077
Fax 404-623-5568

Mini-Wright™ Low Range Peak Flow Meter PF-240X

Same as PF-240 but in a plastic tube, no molded case
Available from:
Armstrong Medical Industries, Inc.
375 Knightsbridge Pkwy. (APD)
PO Box 700 (APD)
Lincolnshire, IL 60069
800-323-4220
In IL 708-913-0101
Fax 708-913-0138
Western States 800-442-6991
Western States Fax 619-535-0525

mini-Wright™ Peak Flow Meter PF-239X

Same as PF-239 but in a plastic tube, no molded case
Available from:
Armstrong Medical Industries, Inc.
375 Knightsbridge Pkwy. (APD)
PO Box 700 (APD)
Lincolnshire, IL 60069
800-323-4220
In IL 708-913-0101
Fax 708-913-0138
Western States 800-442-6991
Western States Fax 619-535-0525

Personal Best™ Low Range Peak Flow Meterz

HealthScan meter with accuracy better than plus or minus 5%; low range 50 to 390 liters per minute; impact resistant, hinged cover folds for a self-contained design for travel; oval mouthpiece; patient record chart; dishwasher safe; 6.5"x2"x.8"; 3 oz.
Available from:
Allergy Asthma Technology
4151 N. Kedzie (APD)
PO Box 18398 (APD)
Chicago, IL 60618
800-621-5545
312-465-8020
Fax 312-465-7619

Asthma Resources Directory

Respiratory Aids

Personal Best™ Peak Flow Meter

HealthScan meter with accuracy better than plus or minus 5%; 90 to 810 liters per minutes; impact resistant, hinged cover folds for a self-contained design for travel; oval mouthpiece; patient record chart; dishwasher safe; 6.5"x2"x.8"; 3 oz.
Available from:
Allergy Asthma Technology
4151 N. Kedzie (APD)
PO Box 18398 (APD)
Chicago, IL 60618
800-621-5545
312-465-8020
Fax 312-465-7619
and:
Allergy Control Products, Inc.
96 Danbury Rd. (APD)
PO Box 793 (APD)
Ridgefield, CT 06877
800-422-DUST (3878)
203-438-9580
Fax 203-431-8963
and:
Allergy Supply Co., Inc. The
11994 Star Court (APD)
Herndon, VA 22071
800-323-6744
Metropolitan DC 703-391-2011
Fax 703-391-2014
BBS 703-521-0638
and:
Allergy-Asthma Shopper™
PO Box 239 (APD)
Fate, TX 75132
800-447-1100
Fax 903-883-4513

Pocketpeak™ Low Range

Mechanism is a flexible, steel vane that bends with exhaled flow rate; accurate within 10%; 50 to 400 liters per minute; integral mouthpiece storage for adult/pediatric mouthpiece; diary booklet; finger hold and thumb rest; zone labels; dishwasher safe; non-prescription; 1-1/2 oz.
Available from:
Ferraris Medical, Inc.

9681 Wagner Rd. (APD)
PO Box 344 (APD)
Holland, NY 14080
800-724-7929
716-537-2391
Fax 716-537-9151

Pocketpeak™ Universal Range

Mechanism is a flexible, steel vane that bends with exhaled flow rate; accurate within 10%; 50 to 720 liters per minute; integral mouthpiece storage for adult/pediatric mouthpiece; diary booklet; finger hold and thumb rest; zone labels; dishwasher safe; non-prescription; 1-1/2 oz.
Available from:
Allergy Asthma Technology
4151 N. Kedzie (APD)
PO Box 18398 (APD)
Chicago, IL 60618
800-621-5545
312-465-8020
Fax 312-465-7619
and:
Ferraris Medical, Inc.
9681 Wagner Rd. (APD)
PO Box 344 (APD)
Holland, NY 14080
800-724-7929
716-537-2391
Fax 716-537-9151

Pulmo-Graph Peak Flow Monitor 580AM

Standard adult range, 50 to 750 liters per minute; resusable mouthpiece and daily record card; accuracy better than plus or minus 5%; 2.6 oz.; 2.25"x7.5"x1.5"
Available from:
Sunrise Medical/DeVilbiss, Inc.
PO Box 635 (APD)
Somerset, PA 15501-0635
800-DeV-1988 (338-1988)
814-443-4881
Fax 800-345-2202
In Canada 705-728-5522

Asthma Resources Directory

Respiratory Aids

Pulmo-Graph Peak Flow Monitor 580PM

Low range, pediatric monitor, 0 to 280 liters per minute; resurable mouth piece and daily record card; accuracy better than plus or minus 5%; 2.6 oz.; 2.25"x7.5"x1.5"
Available from:
Sunrise Medical/DeVilbiss, Inc.
PO Box 635 (APD)
Somerset, PA 15501-0635
800-DeV-1988 (338-1988)
814-443-4881
Fax 800-345-2202
In Canada 705-728-5522

Pulmograph Low Range Peak Flow Meter

Better than plus or minus 5% accuracy; 0 to 280 liters per minute; recording chart; 2.6 oz.
Available from:
Allergy Supply Co., Inc. The
11994 Star Court (APD)
Herndon, VA 22071
800-323-6744
Metropolitan DC 703-391-2011
Fax 703-391-2014
BBS 703-521-0638

Spir-O-Flow

Dual scale for standard (60 to 780 liters/min), low range (35 to 385 liters/min), measurements; mouthpiece adapter acccomodates regular, pediatric disposable mouthpieces; dishwasher safe; instructions, mouthpieces, record chart, pouch; 2.7 oz.
Available from:
Spirometrics, Inc.
415 Rodman Rd. (APD)
Auburn, ME 04210
800-767-0004

SpiroFlow

Dual scale for standard and low range measurements; 60 to 780 liters per minute and 35 to 385 liters per minute; mouthpiece adaptor for adult and pediatric disposable mouthpieces; dishwasher safe; 2.7 oz.
Available from:
CDX Corporation
2 Charles St. (APD)
Providence, RI 02904-9915
800-245-9949
401-274-9518
Fax 401-274-9503

Standard FlowMeter

Measures 60 to 600 liters per minute flow settings; removable mouthpiece; flow tab; whistle casing
Available from:
Biotrine Corp.
52 Dragon Ct. (APD)
Woburn, MA 01801
617-935-8844

The PEAK™ Pediatric

For younger children; dishwasher safe; bright green with colorful stickers
Available from:
A-Plus Allergy Equipment & Supply
8325 Regis Way (APD)
Los Angeles, CA 90045-2646
Orders 800-86-ALLER (862-5537)
310-337-7468
Fax 310-337-1971
and:
Allergy Control Products, Inc.
96 Danbury Rd. (APD)
PO Box 793 (APD)
Ridgefield, CT 06877
800-422-DUST (3878)
203-438-9580
Fax 203-431-8963

The PEAK™

For adults and older children; dishwasher safe
Available from:
A-Plus Allergy Equipment & Supply
8325 Regis Way (APD)
Los Angeles, CA 90045-2646
Orders 800-86-ALLER (862-5537)
310-337-7468
Fax 310-337-1971
and:

Asthma Resources Directory

Respiratory Aids

Allergy Control Products, Inc.
96 Danbury Rd. (APD)
PO Box 793 (APD)
Ridgefield, CT 06877
800-422-DUST (3878)
203-438-9580
Fax 203-431-8963

Truzone™ Peak Flow Meter

Customize meter with red, yellow, and green color strips; measures on visible indicator
Available from:
Allergy & Asthma Network/
Mothers of Asthmatics, Inc.
3554 Chain Bridge Rd. Ste 200 (APD)
Fairfax, VA 22030-2709
Orders 800-878-4403
703-385-4403
Fax 703-352-4354

Vitalograph™ High Range Peak Flow Monitor

Portable; measures up to 750 liters per minute; patient record chart; accuracy better than plus or minus 5%; 2.6 oz.
Available from:
Absolute Environmental's Allergy Store
2615 S. University Dr. (APD)
Davie, FL 33328
Nationwide 800-771-ACHOO (2246)
In FL 800-329-3773
Broward 305-472-3773
Fax 305-474-0133
and:
Allergy & Asthma Network/
Mothers of Asthmatics, Inc.
3554 Chain Bridge Rd. Ste 200 (APD)
Fairfax, VA 22030-2709
Orders 800-878-4403
703-385-4403
Fax 703-352-4354
and:
Allergy Asthma Technology
4151 N. Kedzie (APD)
PO Box 18398 (APD)
Chicago, IL 60618
800-621-5545
312-465-8020

Fax 312-465-7619
and:
HealthScan Products, Inc.
908 Pompton Ave. (APD)
Cedar Grove, NJ 07009-1292
800-962-1266
In NJ 201-857-3414
and:
Vitalograph®
8347 Quivira Rd. (APD)
Lenexa, KS 66215
800-255-6626
913-888-4221
Fax 913-888-4259

Vitalograph™ Low Range Peak Flow Monitor

Patient record chart; measures up to 260 liters per minute; portable, for children and individuals with lower capacity; accuracy better than plus or minus 5%; 2.6 oz.
Available from:
Absolute Environmental's Allergy Store
2615 S. University Dr. (APD)
Davie, FL 33328
Nationwide 800-771-ACHOO (2246)
In FL 800-329-3773
Broward 305-472-3773
Fax 305-474-0133
and:
Allergy & Asthma Network/
Mothers of Asthmatics, Inc.
3554 Chain Bridge Rd. Ste 200 (APD)
Fairfax, VA 22030-2709
Orders 800-878-4403
703-385-4403
Fax 703-352-4354
and:
Allergy Asthma Technology
4151 N. Kedzie (APD)
PO Box 18398 (APD)
Chicago, IL 60618
800-621-5545
312-465-8020
Fax 312-465-7619
and:
Vitalograph®
8347 Quivira Rd. (APD)
Lenexa, KS 66215

Asthma Resources Directory

Respiratory Aids

800-255-6626
913-888-4221
Fax 913-888-4259

VMX Mini-Log™

Logs patient data for computer recall on supplied MS-DOS PC software and records PEF with range of 0 to 800 lpm; accurate to plus or minus 5%; disposable cardboard mouthpieces
Available from:
Clement Clark, Inc.
3128-D E. 17th Ave. (APD)
Columbus, OH 43219
800-848-8923
614-478-2777
Fax 614-478-2622

Wright® Professional Peak Flow Meter PF-286

For hospitals, clinics, and professional use; adult and pediatric sterilizable mouthpieces; disposable mouthpieces; spare filters; rotating vane with attached indicator; dual scale in dial face; outer ring original calibration scale in black; inner scale in red calibrated per the 1991 recommended technical standards
Available from:
Armstrong Medical Industries, Inc.
375 Knightsbridge Pkwy. (APD)
PO Box 700 (APD)
Lincolnshire, IL 60069
800-323-4220
In IL 708-913-0101
Fax 708-913-0138
Western States 800-442-6991
Western States Fax 619-535-0525
and:
Clement Clark, Inc.
3128-D E. 17th Ave. (APD)
Columbus, OH 43219
800-848-8923
614-478-2777
Fax 614-478-2622
and:
Ferraris Medical, Inc.
9681 Wagner Rd. (APD)

PO Box 344 (APD)
Holland, NY 14080
800-724-7929
716-537-2391
Fax 716-537-9151

ADAPTAORS/EXTENDERS

Aerochamber® Inhaler

Tube-shaped chamber holds aerosol drug particles coming from metered dost inhaler; eliminates timing of inhalation with medication release; enhances medication delivery with metered dose inhalers; FloSignal whistle warns against breathing in too quickly; washable pediatric face mask; one-way movement of medication valve
Available from:
Allergy Asthma Technology
4151 N. Kedzie (APD)
PO Box 18398 (APD)
Chicago, IL 60618
800-621-5545
312-465-8020
Fax 312-465-7619
and:
Allergy Supply Co., Inc. The
11994 Star Court (APD)
Herndon, VA 22071
800-323-6744
Metropolitan DC 703-391-2011
Fax 703-391-2014
BBS 703-521-0638
and:
American Allergy Supply
PO Box 722022 (APD)
Houston, TX 77272-2022
800-321-1096
713-995-6110
and:
Immunization Alert®
IMSWORLD Publications, Ltd.
York House
37 Queen Square (APD)
London WC1N 3BL
England
and:
Monaghan Medical Corp.

97

Asthma Resources Directory

Respiratory Aids

PO Box 978 (APD)
Plattsburgh, NY 12901
800-833-9653
In NY 518-561-7330
and:
Pulmonary Paper, The
PO Box 877 (APD)
Ormand Beach, FL 32175
800-950-3698
904-673-7501
Fax 904-673-5044

Azmacort® Inhaler
Built-in aerosol spacer device
telescopes; minimizers need for
coordinating inhalation with
medication release; enhances
medication delivery with metered dose
inhalers
Available from:
Rhone-Poulenc Rorer Pharmaceuticals,
Inc.
500 Arcola Rd. (APD)
PO Box 1200 (APD)
Collegeville, PA 19426-0107
215-454-8000

Brethancer®
Spacer is a medication reservoir to
facilitate inhalation of medication; does
not require coordination of breathing
with medication release for proper
medication delivery; enhances
medication delivery with metered dose
inhalers;
Available from:
Geigy Pharmaceuticals
Div. CIBA-GEIGY Corp.
Ardsley, NY 10502
201-277-5000

Inhal-Aid®
Collecting chamber for medication;
float incentive feature for children to
simplify use of metered dose inhalant
systems; does not require coordination
of breathing with medication release;
enhances medication delivery with
metered dose inhalers
Available from:

Allergy Asthma Technology
4151 N. Kedzie (APD)
PO Box 18398 (APD)
Chicago, IL 60618
800-621-5545
312-465-8020
Fax 312-465-7619
and:
Key Pharmaceuticals, Inc.
Galloping Hill Rd. (APD)
Kenilworth, NJ 07033
800-222-7579
In NJ 908-558-4000

InspirEase™
Mouthpiece fits most metered dose
enhaler systems; whistles if inhale too
fast; universal mouthpiece; replaceable
reservoir bags; enhances medication
delivery with metered dose inhalers;
does not rrequire coordination of
breathing with medication release;
carrying case
Available from:
Allergy Asthma Technology
4151 N. Kedzie (APD)
PO Box 18398 (APD)
Chicago, IL 60618
800-621-5545
312-465-8020
Fax 312-465-7619
and:
Allergy Asthma Technology
4151 N. Kedzie (APD)
PO Box 18398 (APD)
Chicago, IL 60618
800-621-5545
312-465-8020
Fax 312-465-7619
and:
Allergy Supply Co., Inc. The
11994 Star Court (APD)
Herndon, VA 22071
800-323-6744
Metropolitan DC 703-391-2011
Fax 703-391-2014
BBS 703-521-0638
and:
Key Pharmaceuticals, Inc.
Galloping Hill Rd. (APD)

Asthma Resources Directory

Respiratory Aids

Kenilworth, NJ 07033
800-222-7579
In NJ 908-558-4000

Maxair® Autohaler
Inhalation device automatically releases the correct dose of medication upon inhalation; no need to coordinate breathing with medication release; enhances medication delivery with metered dose inhalers
Available from:
3M Company
PO Box 33275 (APD)
St. Paul, MN 55133-3275
3M Center Bldg.(APD)
St. Paul, MN 55144-1000
Medical information 800-328-0255
Medical information local 612-736-4930
Customer service 800-423-5197
Outside CA 800-423-5146
In CA 818-341-1300

OptiHaler®
Spacer system by HealthScan for enhanced medication delivery with metered dose inhalers; aerosol medication particles mix with moving stream of air in a holding chamber before inhalation where larger particles are filtered out; does not require coordination of breathing with medication release; built-in canister holder; children, adults
Available from:
Allergy Asthma Technology
4151 N. Kedzie (APD)
PO Box 18398 (APD)
Chicago, IL 60618
800-621-5545
312-465-8020
Fax 312-465-7619
and:
Allergy Clean Environments
501 Station Ave. (APD)
Haddon Heights, NJ 08035
800-882-4110
In NJ 609-546-1101
Fax 609-546-1466

URL:
http:\\WWW.infomall.com\allergy.html
and:
Allergy Supply Co., Inc. The
11994 Star Court (APD)
Herndon, VA 22071
800-323-6744
Metropolitan DC 703-391-2011
Fax 703-391-2014
BBS 703-521-0638
and:
Allergy-Asthma Shopper™
PO Box 239 (APD)
Fate, TX 75132
800-447-1100
Fax 903-883-4513
and:
HealthScan Products, Inc.
908 Pompton Ave. (APD)
Cedar Grove, NJ 07009-1292
800-962-1266
In NJ 201-857-3414

Pari-Boy® Jet Nebulizer Bowl
Reservoir for intermittent therapy with compressor nebulizers; does not require coordination of breathing with medication release; enhances medication delivery with metered dose inhalers
Available from:
Dura Pharmaceuticals, Inc.
PO Box 2209 (APD)
Ramona, CA 92065-0938
800-231-3195
In CA 619-789-6840

NEBULIZERS
Bronkometer® Pocket Nebulizer
Available from:
Winthrop Pharmaceuticals
Distributed by Winthrop-Breon
Laboratories
Div. of Sterling Drug, Inc.
90 Park Ave. (APD)
New York, NY 10016
212-907-2000

Asthma Resources Directory

Respiratory Aids

DeVilbiss Aerosonic 5000D

Delivers 97% medication as particles between 1 and 3 micron up to 0.5 ml per minute; includes battery pack; reusable circuit; rechargeable battery, wall outlet, or car cigarette lighter; 2-3/4 lbs.
Available from:
Allergy Supply Co., Inc. The
11994 Star Court (APD)
Herndon, VA 22071
800-323-6744
Metropolitan DC 703-391-2011
Fax 703-391-2014
BBS 703-521-0638
and:
Sunrise Medical/DeVilbiss, Inc.
PO Box 635 (APD)
Somerset, PA 15501-0635
800-DeV-1988 (338-1988)
814-443-4881
Fax 800-345-2202
In Canada 705-728-5522

DeVilbiss AeroSonic

Nebuilizes medication so 97% of particles are between 1 and 3 micron in volumes up to .5 ml per minute; mouthpiece with check valve and adapter; rechargeable battery; automatic shut-off; 5"x5-1/4"x2-1/4"; controlling unit, chamber assembly, carrying case; AC/DC adapter/charger, DC power cord; wall outlet, or car cigarette lighter; 2-1/2 lbs.
Available from:
Allergy Supply Co., Inc. The
11994 Star Court (APD)
Herndon, VA 22071
800-323-6744
Metropolitan DC 703-391-2011
Fax 703-391-2014
BBS 703-521-0638
and:
Sunrise Medical/DeVilbiss, Inc.
PO Box 635 (APD)
Somerset, PA 15501-0635
800-DeV-1988 (338-1988)
814-443-4881
Fax 800-345-2202

In Canada 705-728-5522

DeVilbiss Medication Nebulizer

Includes nebuilizer, medicine cup, 7' tubing, T-connector, and mouthpiece
Available from:
Allergy Supply Co., Inc. The
11994 Star Court (APD)
Herndon, VA 22071
800-323-6744
Metropolitan DC 703-391-2011
Fax 703-391-2014
BBS 703-521-0638
and:
Sunrise Medical/DeVilbiss, Inc.
PO Box 635 (APD)
Somerset, PA 15501-0635
800-DeV-1988 (338-1988)
814-443-4881
Fax 800-345-2202
In Canada 705-728-5522

DeVilbiss Nebulizer 646

T-piece enables patient to leave nebulizer in mouth while exhaling; comes with tubing, activator valve, mouthpiece and extra jet
Model 644 for use with mask
Available from:
Sunrise Medical/DeVilbiss, Inc.
PO Box 635 (APD)
Somerset, PA 15501-0635
800-DeV-1988 (338-1988)
814-443-4881
Fax 800-345-2202
In Canada 705-728-5522

DeVilbiss Pocket Nebulizer 45

Portable nebulizer with squeezable rubber bulb, medication cup; break-resistant; Lexan® plastic; includes mouthpiece, extra jet, bulb
Available from:
Allergy Asthma Technology
4151 N. Kedzie (APD)
PO Box 18398 (APD)
Chicago, IL 60618
800-621-5545
312-465-8020

Allergy Products Directory
Copyrighted. Reproduction Prohibited by Law. 1259 El Camino #254, Menlo Park, CA 94025

Asthma Resources Directory

Respiratory Aids

Fax 312-465-7619
and:
Environtrol® Corp.
PO Box 31313 (APD)
St. Louis, MO 63131
800-423-1982
In St. Louis 314-966-6886
and:
Sunrise Medical/DeVilbiss, Inc.
PO Box 635 (APD)
Somerset, PA 15501-0635
800-DeV-1988 (338-1988)
814-443-4881
Fax 800-345-2202
In Canada 705-728-5522

DeVilbiss Pulmo-Aide®
Compressor/Nebulizer
Enhances delivery of medication
by breaking up medication into fine
particles; medication cup, tubing,
mouthpiece, pneumatic nebulizer;
storage for disposable Pulmo-Neb
nebulizer; optional pediatric aerosol
mask; weighs 7-1/4 lbs.; particle size
range 0.5 to 5 micron; UL listed
Available from:
Absolute Environmental's Allergy Store
2615 S. University Dr. (APD)
Davie, FL 33328
Nationwide 800-771-ACHOO (2246)
In FL 800-329-3773
Broward 305-472-3773
Fax 305-474-0133
and:
Allergy Asthma Technology
4151 N. Kedzie (APD)
PO Box 18398 (APD)
Chicago, IL 60618
800-621-5545
312-465-8020
Fax 312-465-7619
and:
Allergy Control Products, Inc.
96 Danbury Rd. (APD)
PO Box 793 (APD)
Ridgefield, CT 06877
800-422-DUST (3878)
203-438-9580
Fax 203-431-8963

and:
Allergy Supply Co., Inc. The
11994 Star Court (APD)
Herndon, VA 22071
800-323-6744
Metropolitan DC 703-391-2011
Fax 703-391-2014
BBS 703-521-0638
and:
American Allergy Supply
PO Box 722022 (APD)
Houston, TX 77272-2022
800-321-1096
713-995-6110
and:
Environtrol® Corp.
PO Box 31313 (APD)
St. Louis, MO 63131
800-423-1982
In St. Louis 314-966-6886
and:
National Allergy Supply, Inc.
4400 Georgia Hwy. 120 (APD)
PO Box 1658 (APD)
Duluth, GA 30136
800-522-1448
In Atlanta 404-623-8077
Fax 404-623-5568
and:
Sunrise Medical/DeVilbiss, Inc.
PO Box 635 (APD)
Somerset, PA 15501-0635
800-DeV-1988 (338-1988)
814-443-4881
Fax 800-345-2202
In Canada 705-728-5522

DeVilbiss Pulmo-Aide® Traveler®
Compressor/Nebulizer
Portable compressor nebulizer;
particle size .5 to 5 micron; uses
household current or rechargeable
battery, indoors or outdoors; optional
DC adapter/charger; 12V DC power
cord for cigarette lighter; carrying case;
medication cup, mouthpiece or mask;
6.4 lbs.; adapter, 4 lbs.
Available from:
Absolute Environmental's Allergy Store
2615 S. University Dr. (APD)

101

Allergy Products Directory

Copyrighted. Reproduction Prohibited by Law. 1259 El Camino #254, Menlo Park, CA 94025

Asthma Resources Directory

Respiratory Aids

Davie, FL 33328
Nationwide 800-771-ACHOO (2246)
In FL 800-329-3773
Broward 305-472-3773
Fax 305-474-0133
and:
Allergy Asthma Technology
4151 N. Kedzie (APD)
PO Box 18398 (APD)
Chicago, IL 60618
800-621-5545
312-465-8020
Fax 312-465-7619
and:
Allergy Control Products, Inc.
96 Danbury Rd. (APD)
PO Box 793 (APD)
Ridgefield, CT 06877
800-422-DUST (3878)
203-438-9580
Fax 203-431-8963
and:
Allergy Solutions
4909 W. Park Blvd. #169 (APD)
Plano, TX 75093
800-380-SNEEZ (7633)
214-612-4188
Fax 214-985-5573
and:
Allergy Supply Co., Inc. The
11994 Star Court (APD)
Herndon, VA 22071
800-323-6744
Metropolitan DC 703-391-2011
Fax 703-391-2014
BBS 703-521-0638
and:
American Allergy Supply
PO Box 722022 (APD)
Houston, TX 77272-2022
800-321-1096
713-995-6110
and:
Sunrise Medical/DeVilbiss, Inc.
PO Box 635 (APD)
Somerset, PA 15501-0635
800-DeV-1988 (338-1988)
814-443-4881
Fax 800-345-2202
In Canada 705-728-5522

DeVilbiss Pulmo-Mate® Compressor/Nebulizer

Like the Pulmo-Aide® but smaller and more compact; fits into suitcase
Available from:
Absolute Environmental's Allergy Store
2615 S. University Dr. (APD)
Davie, FL 33328
Nationwide 800-771-ACHOO (2246)
In FL 800-329-3773
Broward 305-472-3773
Fax 305-474-0133
and:
Sunrise Medical/DeVilbiss, Inc.
PO Box 635 (APD)
Somerset, PA 15501-0635
800-DeV-1988 (338-1988)
814-443-4881
Fax 800-345-2202
In Canada 705-728-5522

DeVilbiss Pulmo-Neb®

Single patient use, 60-day, disposable nebulizer with mouthpiece or optional adult or pediatric mask; tubing, thumb-valve, mouthpiece, and "T" piece
Available from:
Sunrise Medical/DeVilbiss, Inc.
PO Box 635 (APD)
Somerset, PA 15501-0635
800-DeV-1988 (338-1988)
814-443-4881
Fax 800-345-2202
In Canada 705-728-5522

Fisoneb® Ultrasonic Nebulizer

Continuous flow or on-demand mouthpiece, pediatric, adult masks; compact; hand-held unit; 1 lb.
Available from:
Allergy Asthma Technology
4151 N. Kedzie (APD)
PO Box 18398 (APD)
Chicago, IL 60618
800-621-5545
312-465-8020
Fax 312-465-7619

Asthma Resources Directory

Respiratory Aids

HealthDyne Inspiration™ 323 Nebulizer

Portable aerosol unit with compressor; disposable nebulizer/tubing kit; storage for accessories and medication; optional AC/DC unit with car cigarette lighter adapter; 6 lbs.; 8"x4"x11.5"
Available from:
Absolute Environmental's Allergy Store
2615 S. University Dr. (APD)
Davie, FL 33328
Nationwide 800-771-ACHOO (2246)
In FL 800-329-3773
Broward 305-472-3773
Fax 305-474-0133
and:
Allergy Clean Environments
501 Station Ave. (APD)
Haddon Heights, NJ 08035
800-882-4110
In NJ 609-546-1101
Fax 609-546-1466
URL:
http:\\WWW.infomall.com\allergy.html
and:
Allergy Supply Co., Inc. The
11994 Star Court (APD)
Herndon, VA 22071
800-323-6744
Metropolitan DC 703-391-2011
Fax 703-391-2014
BBS 703-521-0638

HealthDyne Nebulizer #929

Vibration-free aerosol unit
Available from:
Allergy Clean Environments
501 Station Ave. (APD)
Haddon Heights, NJ 08035
800-882-4110
In NJ 609-546-1101
Fax 609-546-1466
URL:
http:\\WWW.infomall.com\allergy.html

Hositak Pediatric Medication Nebulizer (aerosol nebulizer)

Nebulizer, tubing, medicine cup, mask

Available from:
Allergy Supply Co., Inc. The
11994 Star Court (APD)
Herndon, VA 22071
800-323-6744
Metropolitan DC 703-391-2011
Fax 703-391-2014
BBS 703-521-0638

Hospitak Pediatric Medication Nebulizer

Includes nebulizer, medicine, cup, 7' tubing, pediatric aerosol mask
Available from:
Allergy Supply Co., Inc. The
11994 Star Court (APD)
Herndon, VA 22071
800-323-6744
Metropolitan DC 703-391-2011
Fax 703-391-2014
BBS 703-521-0638

Hospitak Tote-A-Neb 1500

Built-in, rechargeable battery; household current or car lighter; compressor, power adaptors, standard nebulizer set; 6 lbs.; carrying case
Available from:
Allergy Supply Co., Inc. The
11994 Star Court (APD)
Herndon, VA 22071
800-323-6744
Metropolitan DC 703-391-2011
Fax 703-391-2014
BBS 703-521-0638
and:
Environtrol® Corp.
PO Box 31313 (APD)
St. Louis, MO 63131
800-423-1982
In St. Louis 314-966-6886

Hospitak Tote-A-Neb Nebulizer 1504

Portable nebuilizer uses household outlet or car cigarette lighter; optional rechargeable battery pack; medication cup, tubing mouthpiece, carrying case, strap; 4 lbs.
Available from:

103

Allergy Products Directory

Copyrighted. Reproduction Prohibited by Law. 1259 El Camino #254, Menlo Park, CA 94025

Asthma Resources Directory

Respiratory Aids

Allergy Asthma Technology
4151 N. Kedzie (APD)
PO Box 18398 (APD)
Chicago, IL 60618
800-621-5545
312-465-8020
Fax 312-465-7619
and:
Allergy Supply Co., Inc. The
11994 Star Court (APD)
Herndon, VA 22071
800-323-6744
Metropolitan DC 703-391-2011
Fax 703-391-2014
BBS 703-521-0638
and:
Environtrol® Corp.
PO Box 31313 (APD)
St. Louis, MO 63131
800-423-1982
In St. Louis 314-966-6886

Hospitak Up-Mist Medication Nebulizer
Aerosol nebulizer, tubing,
medicine cup, T-connector,
mouthpiece
Available from:
Allergy Supply Co., Inc. The
11994 Star Court (APD)
Herndon, VA 22071
800-323-6744
Metropolitan DC 703-391-2011
Fax 703-391-2014
BBS 703-521-0638

Hudson "T" Up-Draft II®
High output nebulizer with
reservoir; 7 ft. tubing, 6 ft. flex tubing,
mouothpiece, and t-piece
Available from:
Sunrise Medical/DeVilbiss, Inc.
PO Box 635 (APD)
Somerset, PA 15501-0635
800-DeV-1988 (338-1988)
814-443-4881
Fax 800-345-2202
In Canada 705-728-5522

Inspiration 323
Compact for travel; comes with
disposable nebuilizer-tubing kit;
household outlet or optional car
cigarette lighter adaptor cord
Available from:
Absolute Environmental's Allergy Store
2615 S. University Dr. (APD)
Davie, FL 33328
Nationwide 800-771-ACHOO (2246)
In FL 800-329-3773
Broward 305-472-3773
Fax 305-474-0133

Marquest #3017 Medication Nebulizer
Includes nebulizer, medicine cup,
7' tubing, T-connector, mouthpiece;
nebuilizers from 0 to 90 o angle
Available from:
Allergy Supply Co., Inc. The
11994 Star Court (APD)
Herndon, VA 22071
800-323-6744
Metropolitan DC 703-391-2011
Fax 703-391-2014
BBS 703-521-0638

Medi-Mist Nebulizer
Compressor-driven; storage
container with handle; 7 lbs.
Available from:
Allergy Supply Co., Inc. The
11994 Star Court (APD)
Herndon, VA 22071
800-323-6744
Metropolitan DC 703-391-2011
Fax 703-391-2014
BBS 703-521-0638
and:
Mountain Medical Equipment, Inc.
10488 W. Centennial Rd. (APD)
Littleton, CO 80127
800-525-8950
In CO 518-561-7330

Micro-Whisper Compressor Nebulizer
Portable 12 volt DC compressor;
nebulizes 3cc in 8 to 16 mins.; cup

Allergy Products Directory

Copyrighted. Reproduction Prohibited by Law.1259 El Camino #254, Menlo Park, CA 94025

Asthma Resources Directory

Respiratory Aids

holds nebulizer; recessed controls; weighs 1.75 lbs.; 4.5"x2.5"x3.5"; UL approved; 12 volt DC operation; carrying case, lighter adaptor, wall transformer, nebulizer and cup, "T" piece, mouthpiece, face mask, oxygen tubing, aluminum housing
Available from:
Medisonic U.S.A., Inc.
9600 Main St. (APD)
Clarence, NY 14031
716-759-7213
Fax 716-759-7215

MicroSonic II Medication Inhaler
Incorporates 0 to 10 lpm air source; provides air to the medication vial to deliver through aerosol mask for treatment of infants and children; portable; generates up to 3.5 cc per minute of uniform mist; particle size range 1 to 5 micron; aerosol mask; reusable medication cup; electronics monitor patient demand and unit's fluid level; 4.5"x2.5"x1.75", weighs under 12 oz.; 12 volts UL listed 110 volt AC/DC adaptor, 12 volt cigarette lighter adaptor, carrying case; completion signal
Available from:
Medisonic U.S.A., Inc.
9600 Main St. (APD)
Clarence, NY 14031
716-759-7213
Fax 716-759-7215

MicroSonic Medication Inhaler
Portable; generates up to 3.5 cc per minute of uniform mist; particle size range 1 to 5 micron; aerosol mask; reusable medication cup; electronics monitor patient demand and unit's fluid level; 4.5"x2.5"x1.75", weighs under 12 oz.; 12 volts UL listed 110 volt AC/DC adaptor, 12 volt cigarette lighter adaptor, carrying case; completion signal
Available from:
Medisonic U.S.A., Inc.
9600 Main St. (APD)

Clarence, NY 14031
716-759-7213
Fax 716-759-7215

Microstat™
Portable ultrasonic nebuilizer works on sound waves; microprocessor selects frequency and voltage, availability of medication in bowl, battery status; optional 220V AC removable/rechargeable battery, wall outlet, car cigarette lighter; carrying case, accessories; 2-3/4 lbs.
Available from:
Allergy Supply Co., Inc. The
11994 Star Court (APD)
Herndon, VA 22071
800-323-6744
Metropolitan DC 703-391-2011
Fax 703-391-2014
BBS 703-521-0638
and:
Mountain Medical Equipment, Inc.
10488 W. Centennial Rd. (APD)
Littleton, CO 80127
800-525-8950
In CO 518-561-7330

MiniMax II Ultrasonic Nebulizer
Reusable medication cup handles quantities from .75 ml. to 15 ml.; 12-volt; 4.5"x2.5"x1.75;" 12 oz.
Available from:
Medisonic U.S.A., Inc.
9600 Main St. (APD)
Clarence, NY 14031
716-759-7213
Fax 716-759-7215

Nebuhaler
Plastic, pear-shaped spacer acts as a reservoir for medication; one-way valve; available in Europe
Available from
Astra Pharmaceutical Products, Inc.
50 Otis St. (APD)
Westboro, MA 01581-4428
508-366-1100

Asthma Resources Directory

Respiratory Aids

Omron Comp-Air™

Delivers 30 psi at 12 liters per minute; piston pump with all-metal cylinder; 45 degree angle delivery for reclining treatment; 5 cc medicine cup; 5.5 lbs.
Available from:
Allergy Supply Co., Inc. The
11994 Star Court (APD)
Herndon, VA 22071
800-323-6744
Metropolitan DC 703-391-2011
Fax 703-391-2014
BBS 703-521-0638

Omron Ultra-Air™

Medication is broken into a dense aerosol through ultrasonic vibration; can be hand-held during treatment; 6 ml disposable medicine cup; adjustable positive pressure delivery system; cleanable particle filters; optional rechargeable battery and charger
Available from:
Allergy Supply Co., Inc. The
11994 Star Court (APD)
Herndon, VA 22071
800-323-6744
Metropolitan DC 703-391-2011
Fax 703-391-2014
BBS 703-521-0638

Pari Dura-Neb® 2000

Portable compressor with Pari LC Jet™reusable nebulizer; operate from wall outlet or battery; charged battery delivers 20 to 22 six-minute treatments; warning lights indicate charge level; replaceable filter; carrying case; 5-1/2 lbs.; disposable circuit; optional 220V DC charger adapter for international travel; replacement parts
Available from:
A-Plus Allergy Equipment & Supply
8325 Regis Way (APD)
Los Angeles, CA 90045-2646
Orders 800-86-ALLER (862-5537)
310-337-7468
Fax 310-337-1971

and:
Allergy Asthma Technology
4151 N. Kedzie (APD)
PO Box 18398 (APD)
Chicago, IL 60618
800-621-5545
312-465-8020
Fax 312-465-7619
and:
Allergy Control Products, Inc.
96 Danbury Rd. (APD)
PO Box 793 (APD)
Ridgefield, CT 06877
800-422-DUST (3878)
203-438-9580
Fax 203-431-8963
and:
Allergy Supply Co., Inc. The
11994 Star Court (APD)
Herndon, VA 22071
800-323-6744
Metropolitan DC 703-391-2011
Fax 703-391-2014
BBS 703-521-0638
and:
Allergy Supply Co., Inc. The
11994 Star Court (APD)
Herndon, VA 22071
800-323-6744
Metropolitan DC 703-391-2011
Fax 703-391-2014
BBS 703-521-0638
and:
Allergy-Asthma Shopper™
PO Box 239 (APD)
Fate, TX 75132
800-447-1100
Fax 903-883-4513
and:
American Allergy Supply
PO Box 722022 (APD)
Houston, TX 77272-2022
800-321-1096
713-995-6110
and:
Dura Pharmaceuticals, Inc.
PO Box 2209 (APD)
Ramona, CA 92065-0938
800-231-3195
In CA 619-789-6840

Asthma Resources Directory

Respiratory Aids

and:
National Allergy Supply, Inc.
4400 Georgia Hwy. 120 (APD)
PO Box 1658 (APD)
Duluth, GA 30136
800-522-1448
In Atlanta 404-623-8077
Fax 404-623-5568

Pari LC Jet +™ Nebulizer

Reusable, easy to clean, Pari LC Jet +™ nebulizer provides breath-controlled nebulization with to increase medication delivery to the lower airways and reduce treatment time; attachments, including 7' tubing, mouthpiece; dishwasher safe; replacement parts
Available from:
A-Plus Allergy Equipment & Supply
8325 Regis Way (APD)
Los Angeles, CA 90045-2646
Orders 800-86-ALLER (862-5537)
310-337-7468
Fax 310-337-1971
and:
Allergy & Asthma Network/
Mothers of Asthmatics, Inc.
3554 Chain Bridge Rd. Ste 200 (APD)
Fairfax, VA 22030-2709
Orders 800-878-4403
703-385-4403
Fax 703-352-4354

Pari LC Jet™ Nebulizer

Reusable aerosolizer to increase medication delivery to the lower airways and reduce treatment time; breath-controlled nebulization; includes medicine cup, external air filter, 7' tubing, mouthpiece; dishwasher safe; optional interrupt valve and pediatric mask; replacement parts
Available from:
Allergy & Asthma Network/
Mothers of Asthmatics, Inc.
3554 Chain Bridge Rd. Ste 200 (APD)
Fairfax, VA 22030-2709
Orders 800-878-4403

703-385-4403
Fax 703-352-4354
and:
Allergy Asthma Technology
4151 N. Kedzie (APD)
PO Box 18398 (APD)
Chicago, IL 60618
800-621-5545
312-465-8020
Fax 312-465-7619
and:
Allergy Supply Co., Inc. The
11994 Star Court (APD)
Herndon, VA 22071
800-323-6744
Metropolitan DC 703-391-2011
Fax 703-391-2014
BBS 703-521-0638
and:
Allergy-Asthma Shopper™
PO Box 239 (APD)
Fate, TX 75132
800-447-1100
Fax 903-883-4513
and:
Dura Pharmaceuticals, Inc.
PO Box 2209 (APD)
Ramona, CA 92065-0938
800-231-3195
In CA 619-789-6840
and:
National Allergy Supply, Inc.
4400 Georgia Hwy. 120 (APD)
PO Box 1658 (APD)
Duluth, GA 30136
800-522-1448
In Atlanta 404-623-8077
Fax 404-623-5568

Pari ProNeb™ Compressor

Light weight compressor with Pari LC Jet +™ reusable nebulizer and attachments; reduces treatment time; built-in thermal protection; operates from wall outlet
Available from:
Allergy Asthma Technology
4151 N. Kedzie (APD)
PO Box 18398 (APD)
Chicago, IL 60618

107

Asthma Resources Directory

Respiratory Aids

800-621-5545
312-465-8020
Fax 312-465-7619
and:
Allergy Control Products, Inc.
96 Danbury Rd. (APD)
PO Box 793 (APD)
Ridgefield, CT 06877
800-422-DUST (3878)
203-438-9580
Fax 203-431-8963
and:
Allergy-Asthma Shopper™
PO Box 239 (APD)
Fate, TX 75132
800-447-1100
Fax 903-883-4513
and:
American Allergy Supply
PO Box 722022 (APD)
Houston, TX 77272-2022
800-321-1096
713-995-6110
and:
National Allergy Supply, Inc.
4400 Georgia Hwy. 120 (APD)
PO Box 1658 (APD)
Duluth, GA 30136
800-522-1448
In Atlanta 404-623-8077
Fax 404-623-5568

Porta-Sonic Portable Nebulizer

Ultrasonic nebulizer for use while traveling; 2-3/4 lbs. with battery; 97% particles between 1 and 3 micron; to 0.5 ml per minute; recharge from wall outlet or car cigarette lighter
Available from:
Sunrise Medical/DeVilbiss, Inc.
PO Box 635 (APD)
Somerset, PA 15501-0635
800-DeV-1988 (338-1988)
814-443-4881
Fax 800-345-2202
In Canada 705-728-5522

Pulmo-Sonic Nebulizer

Ultrasonic nebulizer for fine mist; 4.5 lbs.

Available from:
Sunrise Medical/DeVilbiss, Inc.
PO Box 635 (APD)
Somerset, PA 15501-0635
800-DeV-1988 (338-1988)
814-443-4881
Fax 800-345-2202
In Canada 705-728-5522

Puritan Bennett Medication Nebulizer (aerosol nebulizer)

Nebulizer, tubing, medicine cup, T-connector, mouthpiece
Available from:
Allergy Supply Co., Inc. The
11994 Star Court (APD)
Herndon, VA 22071
800-323-6744
Metropolitan DC 703-391-2011
Fax 703-391-2014
BBS 703-521-0638

Puritan Bennett Pediatric Medication Nebulizer

Medicine cup, 7 ft. tubing; pediatric aerosol mask
Available from:
Allergy Supply Co., Inc. The
11994 Star Court (APD)
Herndon, VA 22071
800-323-6744
Metropolitan DC 703-391-2011
Fax 703-391-2014
BBS 703-521-0638

Spiral 3612 Portable Ultrasonic Drug Inhaler

Portable, 12 volt operation; reusable medication cup holds up to 25 ml. medication; reusable cups; air fan assisst delivers particles to aerosol mask for children and infants; particle size range 1 to 5 micron; 6"x6"x2", 2.5 lbs.; batteries built in, aluminum, 110 volt AC/DC adaptor, 12 volt cigarette lighter adaptor, carrying case, air flow assist assembly, accessories
Available from:
Medisonic U.S.A., Inc.
9600 Main St. (APD)

Asthma Resources Directory

Respiratory Aids

Clarence, NY 14031
716-759-7213
Fax 716-759-7215

Spiral Mark V Portable Ultrasonic Drug Inhaler

Portable, temperature controlled, medication cups, air-assist for children; 25 mls. capacity; electronics monitor patient demand and unit's fluid level; 12 volt DC; built-in charger, batteries, 110 volt AC/DC adaptor, 12 volt cigarette lighter adaptor, carrying case; 5"x5"x2" deep; weighs 2.5 lbs.
Available from:
Medisonic U.S.A., Inc.
9600 Main St. (APD)
Clarence, NY 14031
716-759-7213
Fax 716-759-7215

Travel Adaptor

A/C D/C Unit with cigarette lighter adaptor cord for HealthDyne Inspiration™323 Nebulizer
Available from:
Absolute Environmental's Allergy Store
2615 S. University Dr. (APD)
Davie, FL 33328
Nationwide 800-771-ACHOO (2246)
In FL 800-329-3773
Broward 305-472-3773
Fax 305-474-0133

Whisper Compressor Nebulizer

Portable, nebulizes 3cc in 8 to 16 mins.; cup holds nebulizer; recessed controls; weighs 3.5 lbs.; 7.5"x2.5"x4.25"; UL approved; built-in 12 volt rechargeable battery; carrying case, lighter adaptor, wall transformer, nebulizer and cup, "T" piece, mouthpiece, face mask, oxygen tubing, aluminum housing
Available from:
Medisonic U.S.A., Inc.
9600 Main St. (APD)
Clarence, NY 14031
716-759-7213
Fax 716-759-7215

INCENTIVE EXERCISERS

Breather,™ The

Separately adjustable inhalation and exhalation resistance; exhalation resistance mimics pursed-lip breathing; after removing rubber diaphragm, can clean in boiling water or disinfect
Available from:
PAL Medical, Inc
235 S. Maitland Ave. #214 (APD)
Maitland, FL 32751
800-873-0773
407-539-1302
Fax 407-539-0775

Coach Incentive Exerciser

Inspiratory flow guide; volume indicator; one-way valve; encourages slow inhalation; impact-resistant plastic
Available from:
Allergy Supply Co., Inc. The
11994 Star Court (APD)
Herndon, VA 22071
800-323-6744
Metropolitan DC 703-391-2011
Fax 703-391-2014
BBS 703-521-0638

Coach Jr.

Colorful design; bubblegum flavor, fragrance; game to monitor progress; impact-resistant plastic
Available from:
Allergy Supply Co., Inc. The
11994 Star Court (APD)
Herndon, VA 22071
800-323-6744
Metropolitan DC 703-391-2011
Fax 703-391-2014
BBS 703-521-0638

Pflex Assess Exerciser

Adjustable resistance dial, six settings; readout dial
Available from:
Allergy Asthma Technology
4151 N. Kedzie (APD)

Asthma Resources Directory

Respiratory Aids

PO Box 18398 (APD)
Chicago, IL 60618
800-621-5545
312-465-8020
Fax 312-465-7619
and:
Allergy Supply Co., Inc. The
11994 Star Court (APD)
Herndon, VA 22071
800-323-6744
Metropolitan DC 703-391-2011
Fax 703-391-2014
BBS 703-521-0638

Pflex Inspiratory Trainer
Readout dial; six resistance settings
Available from:
Allergy Supply Co., Inc. The
11994 Star Court (APD)
Herndon, VA 22071
800-323-6744
Metropolitan DC 703-391-2011
Fax 703-391-2014
BBS 703-521-0638
and:
Environtrol® Corp.
PO Box 31313 (APD)
St. Louis, MO 63131
800-423-1982
In St. Louis 314-966-6886
and:
Pulmonary Paper, The
PO Box 877 (APD)
Ormand Beach, FL 32175
800-950-3698
904-673-7501
Fax 904-673-5044

SIE Resistive Trainer™
Inhalation against slight resistance
Available from
PAL Medical, Inc.
235 S. Maitland Ave., Ste. 214 (APD)
Maitland, FL 32751
800-873-0773

Threshold®
Inspiratory muscle trainer with constant inspiratory pressure load independent of air flow or breathing rate
Available from:
Vacumetrics
Vacu-Med
4483 McGrath St. #102 (APD)
Ventura, CA 93003
800-235-3333
805-644-7461
Fax 805-654-8759

Voldyne Deep Breather
Measures sustained maximal inspiration to 400 milliliters
Available from:
Allergy Asthma Technology
4151 N. Kedzie (APD)
PO Box 18398 (APD)
Chicago, IL 60618
800-621-5545
312-465-8020
Fax 312-465-7619

AUXILIARY PRODUCTS

Blairex® Broncho Saline
Can dispenses 1 cc metered doses of .9% sodium chloride, sterile normal saline to dilute bronchodilator medications that are nebulized
Available from:
Allergy Asthma Technology
4151 N. Kedzie (APD)
PO Box 18398 (APD)
Chicago, IL 60618
800-621-5545
312-465-8020
Fax 312-465-7619

Control III Germicide
Cold sterilization for respiratory accessories; solution lasts 14 days
Available from:
Allergy Asthma Technology
4151 N. Kedzie (APD)
PO Box 18398 (APD)

Asthma Resources Directory

Respiratory Aids

Chicago, IL 60618
800-621-5545
312-465-8020
Fax 312-465-7619

Devilbiss Blow-Thru Mouthpiece

Mouthpiece accessory for older patients, children
Available from:
Sunrise Medical/DeVilbiss, Inc.
PO Box 635 (APD)
Somerset, PA 15501-0635
800-DeV-1988 (338-1988)
814-443-4881
Fax 800-345-2202
In Canada 705-728-5522

DeVilbiss Compressor AP-50™

Professional use; holds 1000 ml. sterile water; 26 psi at 7 liters per minute; locking pressure gauge regulator; air inlet filter, fan filter, filter grill; carrying handle; carrying case; 12 lbs.10"x9.5"x10.5" (with gooseneck 11.75");
Available from:
Sunrise Medical/DeVilbiss, Inc.
PO Box 635 (APD)
Somerset, PA 15501-0635
800-DeV-1988 (338-1988)
814-443-4881
Fax 800-345-2202
In Canada 705-728-5522

DeVilbiss Model 180 Regulator

Regulates size of nebulized particles by adjustment of baffle above outlet tube; detachable nasal guard restricts devlelopment of undesirable pressure; small and large plain guards for inflation purposes
Available from:
Sunrise Medical/DeVilbiss, Inc.
PO Box 635 (APD)
Somerset, PA 15501-0635
800-DeV-1988 (338-1988)
814-443-4881
Fax 800-345-2202
In Canada 705-728-5522

DeVilbiss Nebulizer Face Mask

Face mask for older patients, children
Available from:
Sunrise Medical/DeVilbiss, Inc.
PO Box 635 (APD)
Somerset, PA 15501-0635
800-DeV-1988 (338-1988)
814-443-4881
Fax 800-345-2202
In Canada 705-728-5522

DeVilbiss Pulmo-Aide® Compressor/Nebulizer 5612M

Compressor connects to car, battery pack or other 12 volt DC source; air displacement is 18 lpm; nebuilizer, tubing, thumb-valve included
Available from:
Sunrise Medical/DeVilbiss, Inc.
PO Box 635 (APD)
Somerset, PA 15501-0635
800-DeV-1988 (338-1988)
814-443-4881
Fax 800-345-2202
In Canada 705-728-5522

DeVilbiss Right-Angle Nebulizer Accessory

Accessory for bedridden patients
Available from:
Sunrise Medical/DeVilbiss, Inc.
PO Box 635 (APD)
Somerset, PA 15501-0635
800-DeV-1988 (338-1988)
814-443-4881
Fax 800-345-2202
In Canada 705-728-5522

Dey-Pak™ Sodium Chloride Solution

Pre-measured saline solutions of 3 ml. vials for nebulizers; two concentrations: .9% and .45% sodium chloride
Available from:
Allergy Asthma Technology
4151 N. Kedzie (APD)
PO Box 18398 (APD)

111

Asthma Resources Directory

Respiratory Aids

Chicago, IL 60618
800-621-5545
312-465-8020
Fax 312-465-7619
and:
Sunrise Medical/DeVilbiss, Inc.
PO Box 635 (APD)
Somerset, PA 15501-0635
800-DeV-1988 (338-1988)
814-443-4881
Fax 800-345-2202
In Canada 705-728-5522

Disposable Aerosol Masks
Used for nebulizer treatments; includes adjustable elastic retaining strap, coupling, built-in metal nose clip
Available from:
Allergy Supply Co., Inc. The
11994 Star Court (APD)
Herndon, VA 22071
800-323-6744
Metropolitan DC 703-391-2011
Fax 703-391-2014
BBS 703-521-0638
and:
Sunrise Medical/DeVilbiss, Inc.
PO Box 635 (APD)
Somerset, PA 15501-0635
800-DeV-1988 (338-1988)
814-443-4881
Fax 800-345-2202
In Canada 705-728-5522

Disposable Pediatric Aerosol Masks
Used for nebulizer treatments; includes adjustable elastic retaining strap, coupling, built-in metal nose clip
Available from:
Allergy Supply Co., Inc. The
11994 Star Court (APD)
Herndon, VA 22071
800-323-6744
Metropolitan DC 703-391-2011
Fax 703-391-2014
BBS 703-521-0638
and:

Sunrise Medical/DeVilbiss, Inc.
PO Box 635 (APD)
Somerset, PA 15501-0635
800-DeV-1988 (338-1988)
814-443-4881
Fax 800-345-2202
In Canada 705-728-5522

NEBU-SOL Saline
Sterile, normal saline for diluting bronchodilator solutions; valve dispenses 1 cc of saline; 300 cc container
Available from:
Allergy Supply Co., Inc. The
11994 Star Court (APD)
Herndon, VA 22071
800-323-6744
Metropolitan DC 703-391-2011
Fax 703-391-2014
BBS 703-521-0638

Pari Pediatric Mask
Mask eases nebulizer use for children; use only with Pari-Jet and Pari LC nebulizer systems
Available from:
Allergy & Asthma Network/
Mothers of Asthmatics, Inc.
3554 Chain Bridge Rd. Ste 200 (APD)
Fairfax, VA 22030-2709
Orders 800-878-4403
703-385-4403
Fax 703-352-4354

PowerStar POW-200
Converter that plugs into car's cigarette lighter for battery power to run nebulizer; also for RV, boat or plane; automatic overload shutdown and recovery; 5"x2.6"x1.7"; 15 oz.
Available from:
Allergy Supply Co., Inc. The
11994 Star Court (APD)
Herndon, VA 22071
800-323-6744
Metropolitan DC 703-391-2011
Fax 703-391-2014
BBS 703-521-0638

112

Asthma Resources Directory

Respiratory Aids

Tubing
Plastic, three-channel, no-cruch supply tubing; 7 ft.
Available from:
Allergy Supply Co., Inc. The
11994 Star Court (APD)
Herndon, VA 22071
800-323-6744
Metropolitan DC 703-391-2011
Fax 703-391-2014
BBS 703-521-0638

Tubing
Plastic, three-channel, no-cruch supply tubing; 25 ft.
Available from:
Allergy Supply Co., Inc. The
11994 Star Court (APD)
Herndon, VA 22071
800-323-6744
Metropolitan DC 703-391-2011
Fax 703-391-2014
BBS 703-521-0638

VentEase
Fits over metered dose inhaler; enables user to squeeze inhaler
Available from:
Allen & Hanburys™
Div. of Glaxo, Inc.
5 Moore Dr. (APD)
Research Triangle Park, NC 27709
919-248-2100
Medical services 919-248-2100

PULMONARY FUNCTION TESTING SYSTEMS

AirWays Respiratory Workstation
Windows with graphical user interface requires no memorized commands; mouse-point to test required; color graphic patient education tutorials, color graphic patient incentives; on-line storage for patient records; full selection of predicted normals
Available from:
Circadian

3942 N. First St. (APD)
San Jose, CA 95134
800-669-7002
408-943-9222
Fax 408-954-1808

CMD/PC-Flow+
Filter disk, volume/time curve and pre/post bronchodilator comparison automatically printed; visual incentive display; accurate to plus or minus 2%; methacholine challenge test; uses IBM compatible computer display
Available from:
Spirometrics, Inc.
415 Rodman Rd. (APD)
Auburn, ME 04210
800-767-0004

Compact II Spirometer
Twenty-five pre-programmed inspiratory and expiratory lung function parameters, including pre and post bronchodilator/provocation tests; back-lit screen, printer; selectable predicted normal values; portable; accurate to plus or minus 3%
Available from:
Vitalograph®
8347 Quivira Rd. (APD)
Lenexa, KS 66215
800-255-6626
913-888-4221
Fax 913-888-4259

Datamite F™
Automatic BTPS correction, pre-post bronchodilator, zero extrapolation; stores FVC, MVV, and B-D tests; waterless; keypad; adult, pediatric, ethnic standards
Available from:
Jones Medical Instrument Co.
200 Windsor Dr. (APD)
Oak Brook, IL 60521
800-323-7336
708-571-1980
Fax 708-571-2023

113

Allergy Products Directory

Copyrighted. Reproduction Prohibited by Law. 1259 El Camino #254, Menlo Park, CA 94025

Asthma Resources Directory

Respiratory Aids

Datamite V® Pulmonaire

Built-in storage for patient data; computer printer; ASCII port for data transmission; communication software for modem transmission to multiple sites or to PC or mainframe; interchangeable sets of predicteds; pediatric and ethnic standards; waterless
Available from:
Jones Medical Instrument Co.
200 Windsor Dr. (APD)
Oak Brook, IL 60521
800-323-7336
708-571-1980
Fax 708-571-2023

Escort Spirometer

Hand-held spirometer with rechargeable battery; no moving parts; calibration, testing, and displaying results on screen; flowhead can be cold sterilized or autoclaved
Available from:
Vitalograph®
8347 Quivira Rd. (APD)
Lenexa, KS 66215
800-255-6626
913-888-4221
Fax 913-888-4259

Flowmate 2500

Prints out test results; visual incentive display; volume/time curve and pre/post bronchodilator comparison automatically printed; calculates 17 indices; LCD prompts; accurate to plus or minus 3%; optional serial output to computers, external printers; 9 lbs.
Available from:
Spirometrics, Inc.
415 Rodman Rd. (APD)
Auburn, ME 04210
800-767-0004

Flowmate Plus 2500+

Prints out test results; visual incentive display; volume/time curve and pre/post bronchodilator comparison automatically printed; calculates 17 indices; methacholine challenge test; LCD prompts; accurate to plus or minus 3%; optional serial output to computers, external printers; 9 lbs.
Available from:
Spirometrics, Inc.
415 Rodman Rd. (APD)
Auburn, ME 04210
800-767-0004

FlowmateLTE

All functions, memory, battery-operated, portable; customized reports printed through parallel port; external filters
Available from:
Spirometrics, Inc.
415 Rodman Rd. (APD)
Auburn, ME 04210
800-767-0004

Puritan Bennett PB100

Portable, with configurable software providing inspiratory/expiratory parameters, pre- and post-medication comparisons, choice of report formats; disposable flow sensors; incentive display and varied motivating tone; rechargeable NiCad battery; reusable patient data memory card; combination charging station/printer modem
Available from:
Puritan-Bennett
900 Springer Dr. (APD)
Lombard, IL 60148-6404
800-255-5444
Regional IL 800-255-6773
Regional GA 404-822-0700
For Home Care 800-248-0890
708-495-5444
Fax 800-755-8075
Fax 708-495-4433

Satellite® Spirometer

Portable, hand-held unit (1 lb.) interfaces with various printers or optional desk unit with printer;

Asthma Resources Directory

Respiratory Aids

internal test storage; LCD display; customized printout; mouthpiece for both inspiratory/expiratory testing; mouthpiece/transducer combination and disposbale measuring system
Available from:
Jones Medical Instrument Co.
200 Windsor Dr. (APD)
Oak Brook, IL 60521
800-323-7336
708-571-1980
Fax 708-571-2023

Satellite/Base Station
Incorporates the portable, hand-held spirometer with the base station; base station functions as recharger, thermal printer, database, and computer interface
Available from:
Jones Medical Instrument Co.
200 Windsor Dr. (APD)
Oak Brook, IL 60521
800-323-7336
708-571-1980
Fax 708-571-2023

SMI I
Pre/post bronchodilator comparison; can be computer integrated; FVD and FEV 1 are compared with norms; checks 7 volume-time parameters; accurate to plus or minus 3%; 12 lbs.
Available from:
Spirometrics, Inc.
415 Rodman Rd. (APD)
Auburn, ME 04210
800-767-0004

SMI III
Operator prompts; keyboard entry; pre/post bronchodilator comparison; prints results, outputs to external printers; automatic calculation of volume/time parameters; accurate to plus or minus 3%; 14 lbs.
Available from:
Spirometrics, Inc.
415 Rodman Rd. (APD)

Auburn, ME 04210
800-767-0004

Spiro 110 MAX
Multiple patient data memory; incentive display; prompts and menu screens; full-function, portable spirometer; reports on 16 diagnostic values; graphs predicted and actual flow loops; cold sterilization; disposable mouthpieces
Available from:
CDX Corporation
2 Charles St. (APD)
Providence, RI 02904-9915
800-245-9949
401-274-9518
Fax 401-274-9503

Spiro 110M
Metric patient values; 220 v/50Hz power supply; prompts and menu screens; full-function, portable spirometer; reports on 16 diagnostic values; graphs predicted and actual flow loops; cold sterilization; disposable mouthpieces
Available from:
CDX Corporation
2 Charles St. (APD)
Providence, RI 02904-9915
800-245-9949
401-274-9518
Fax 401-274-9503

Spiro 110s
Built-in four-color plotter; prompts and menu screens; full-function, portable spirometer; reports on 16 diagnostic values; graphs predicted and actual flow loops; cold sterilization; disposable mouthpieces
Available from:
CDX Corporation
2 Charles St. (APD)
Providence, RI 02904-9915
800-245-9949
401-274-9518
Fax 401-274-9503

Asthma Resources Directory

Respiratory Aids

SpiroLab

Menu-driven software IBM-compatible; customized reports on-screen or printed; prediction quadrant; volume-time curve and pre/post bronchodilator comparison displayed; mouthpiece filter disk; accurate to plus or minus 3%; optional stand
Available from:
Spirometrics, Inc.
415 Rodman Rd. (APD)
Auburn, ME 04210
800-767-0004

Spiromate AS-600

Programmable parameters for challenge test; pharmacologic, cold air, and nonspecific challenges; programmable printout, parallel printer port; calculation of target dosage; data retention while power is off; on screen help; 8.5 lbs.
Available from:
Riko Medical & Scientific Instrument (USA) Corp.
600 Sylvan Ave. (APD)
Englewood Cliffs, NJ 07632
800-222-RIKO (7450)

SpiroNova

Real time display; portable; health screens, work history, trend analysis, management reports; accurate to plus or minus 3%; on-line help
Available from:
CDX Corporation
2 Charles St. (APD)
Providence, RI 02904-9915
800-245-9949
401-274-9518
Fax 401-274-9503

Spirotrac III

Computer-based spirometry system with graphics software; linearized dry wedge-type bellows; 0.04L activation volume; accurate to within plus or minus 0.5%
Available from:
Vitalograph®

8347 Quivira Rd. (APD)
Lenexa, KS 66215
800-255-6626
913-888-4221
Fax 913-888-4259

Survey Spirometers

Standard spirometer is manual operation, calculations made by operator based on direct kymograph tracing reading; water seal or dry seal. Survey II: 10-liter with linear motion potentiometer, 2-speed kymo-graph, water drain; water seal or dry. Survey/PLUS: 10 liter with com-puter interface for spirometry testing, report configuration, interpretation and prediction of results; optional software for provocation or trending
Available from:
Warren E. Collins, Inc.
220 Wood Rd. (APD)
Braintree, MA 02184-2403
800-225-5157
Fax 617-843-4024

SurveyTach Screener

Mobile, high-volume, spirometric screener; protective filter available; cleaned by cold chemical or ethylene oxide techniques; driven by PLUS SQL software
Available from:
Warren E. Collins, Inc.
220 Wood Rd. (APD)
Braintree, MA 02184-2403
800-225-5157
Fax 617-843-4024

Vitalograph S

Linearized dry wedge-type bellows; accurate to plus or mius 0.5%; activation volume 0.04L; inkless stylus
Available from:
Vitalograph®
8347 Quivira Rd. (APD)
Lenexa, KS 66215
800-255-6626
913-888-4221
Fax 913-888-4259

Allergy Products Directory

Copyrighted. Reproduction Prohibited by Law. 1259 El Camino #254, Menlo Park, CA 94025

Asthma Resources Directory
Preparing for Emergencies

EMERGENCIES

If you or a member of your family are involved in an accident, you may have to give accurate, detailed medical information about your health status and medical needs. Problems arise when you are unconscious, are unable to speak, or if the victim is a child, or elderly, or very upset.

Paramedics, ambulance personnel, doctors, emergency room personnel all need to know what your special needs are, especially if you are allergic or asthmatic.

Emergency medical data cards, vials, bracelets, key rings, tags all serve that function. They can communicate for you, including telephone numbers of family, doctors, medical information providers, blood type, allergies. They can allow you to receive more immediate, more appropriate, and safer health care.

Printed cards summarize your medical data, but are not immediately visible. Be sure to carry these cards front and center in your wallet and be sure that the company has an emergency telephone number that operates 24 hours. ID necklaces have room for only a few words. They should also have an emergency 24-hour telephone number with full data access.

Microfiches carry all the information necessary, but need special readers otherwise the information cannot be retrieved. Our listing describes one card which incorporates its own microfiche reader.

PREPARE FOR EMERGENCIES

Ana-Guard™

Treatment for anaphylactic reactions from insect stings, food, drugs, and life-threatening asthma attacks; pre-filled syringe contains two 0.3 ml. doses of epinephrine; barrel marked with 0.1 ml graduations for infants and children under 12 years; prescription required
Available from:
Miles Inc. Pharmaceutical Div.
Miles Allergy Products
(Hollister-Stier)
PO Box 3145 (APD)
3525 N. Regal (APD)
Spokane, WA 99220-3145
800-992-1120
509-489-5656

Ana-Kit®

Contains pre-filled syringe with two 0.3 ml. doses of epinephrine for anaphylactic reactions from insect stings, food, drugs, and life-threatenng asthma attacks; syringe marked for infants and children under 12; chewable antihistamine tablets; 2 alcohol prep pads; tourniquet; carrying case; prescription required
Available from:
Miles Inc. Pharmaceutical Div.
Miles Allergy Products
(Hollister-Stier)
PO Box 3145 (APD)
3525 N. Regal (APD)
Spokane, WA 99220-3145
800-992-1120
509-489-5656

117

Asthma Resources Directory

Preparing for Emergencies

Child's Medical Record

Booklet for entering drug sensitivities, allergies, immunizations (with recommended schedule), illnesses, medications, injuries, operations, dental examinations, and a record of height and weight
Available from:
Child's Medical Record
PO Box 17718
Memphis, TN 38187
901-767-0239

EpiPen Jr.®

Automatically injects correct epinephrine dosage for children; FDA approved for reactions to insect stings, foods, drugs, and exercise-induced anaphylaxis
Available from:
Center Laboratories
35 Channel Dr. (APD)
PO Box 70 (APD)
Port Washington, NY 11050
Customer service 800-223-6837

EpiPen®

Automatically injects correct epinephrine dosage; FDA approved for reactions to insect stings, foods, drugs, and exercised-induced anaphylaxis
Available from:
Center Laboratories
35 Channel Dr. (APD)
PO Box 70 (APD)
Port Washington, NY 11050
Customer service 800-223-6837

Parent Package

For school children with anaphylaxis; 32 page booklet with information about anaphylaxis, guidelines for emergency procedures, overhead transparencies for school personnel, forms for co-operative procedures; literature on adrenaline injection devices; non-functioning injection unit; paypable in Canadian funds
Available from:

Allergy/Asthma Information Assn.
30 Eglinton Ave. W. #750 (APD)
Mississauga, ON L5R 3E7
Canada
905-712-AAIA (2242)
Fax 905-712-2245

Portable Medical Record (MEDPASS)

Lists allergies, allergies to medications; EKG, medications being taken, emergency contact, past history; for corporate subscribers to Global Emergenecy Medical Services; information is maintained online by a 24-hour medical help desk staffed by registered nurses with emergency room experience.
Available from:
Global Emergency Medical Services
2001 Westside Dr. #120
Alpharetta, GA 30201
800-860-1111

COMMUNICATION DURING EMERGENCIES

AT&T Language Line
800-628-8486 fee
For assistance with health language problems

Emergency Identification Sticker

Sticker states name, address, blood type, allergies, emergency telephone contact and insurance carrier; for use on bicycle helmet or bicycle frame
Available from:
Specialized
15130 Concord Cir. (APD)
Morgan Hill, CA 95037
800-688-3883
800-245-3462
and
Specialized Canada
5782 Cypihot St. (APD)
Ville St. Laurent, PQ H4S 1V7
Canada

Asthma Resources Directory
Preparing for Emergencies

and:
Specialized U.K.
Unit D3
Longmed Business Centre
Felstead Rd. (APD)
Eepsom, Surrey KT19 9QN
England

Emergency Medical ID

Laminated, wallet-sized card details medical history on microfilm; your photo can be laminated (and replaced as needed) or slipped into pocket on card for ease of replacement; height, weight, and hair color can be changed as needed
Available from:
EMID
23 Wensley Rd. (APD)
Plainview, NY 11803
516-935-5809

Information Card

Wallet-size card with your medical information; when calling, ask for information desk and then an answer center representative
Available from:
American Medical Assn.
515 N. State St. (APD)
Chicago, IL 60610
312-464-5000
Fax 312-464-4184

Laser Card

For group providers, hospitals, HMO's, group practices.
Laser card holds graphics, x-rays; magnetic stripe or IC chip; lists medical problems, medications and interactions, insurance information, person to notify;
Available from:
Smart Card Systems
15911 Forsythia Cir. (APD)
Del Ray Beach, FL 33484
407-495-2590
Fax 407-243-8740

Lens-Card™

Card with medical information on microfilm with built-in lens; stickers for car or wallet to alert others that you have the card
Available from:
LENSCARD® Systems
7300 Corporate Center Dr. #2C03 (APD)
Miami, FL 33126
PO Box 025491 (APD)
Miami, FL 33102-5491
800-322-3025
In Fl 305-715-3405

Life Alert

Stainless steel or gold fill case contains metal pages with medical data; pendant or bracelet available; up to 50 words for medications, allergies, drug allergy, emergency contact, contact lenses, emergency phone numbers
Available from:
Life Alert
Ste. 112, 7710 5th St SE (APD)
Calgary, AB T2H 2L9
Canada
403-258-0822
Fax 403-242-9132
and
13807 S.E. McLoughlin Blvd. #43 (APD)
Portland, OR 97222

Lifedata Systems

Medical history on microfilm readable by magnifying glass, microscope, or microfiche reader; includes tag for key ring
Available from:
Lifedata Systems, Inc.
PO Box 399 (APD)
Nevada City, CA 95959
800-345-3557

Medic Alert

Metal bracelet or pendant (stainless steel, sterling silver, gold fill)

119

Asthma Resources Directory
Preparing for Emergencies

engraved with medical condition(s), ID number, Medic Alert's emergency hotline number for computerized records
Available from:
Canada Medic-Alert
Affiliate of Medic Alert Foundation
250 Ferrand Dr. (APD)
Don Mills, ON M2C 2T9
Canada
416-696-0267
80-668-1507
and:
Medic Alert Foundation
2323 N. Colorado Ave. (APD)
PO Box 1009 (APD)
Turlock, CA 95381-1009
800-344-3226
800-432-5378
AK, HI 209-668-3333

Medic-Alert

Sports fabric bracelet with medical condition(s), ID number, Medic Alert's emergency hotline number for computerized records
Available from:
Canada Medic-Alert
Affiliate of Medic Alert Foundation
250 Ferrand Dr. (APD)
Don Mills, ON M2C 2T9
Canada
416-696-0267
80-668-1507

Medic-Card

Folding card in plastic case with medical data, including medications, allergies, immunizations, history; emergency notification, insurance, glasses Rx; optional magnet to affix to refrigerator door
Available from:
National Medi-Card Systems
1070 Commerce St. #F (APD)
San Marcos, CA 92069
800-266-1787
In CA 619-744-1787

Medical Alert

Bracelet with wallet card, key tag with wallet card; wallet cards have room for personal identification, social security number, emergency notification, doctor number, blood type, insurance company and medical information
Available from:
Apex™Medical Corp.
800 S. Van Eps Ave. (APD)
Sioux Falls, SD 57104
PO Box 1235 (APD)
Sioux Falls, SD 57101
800-328-2935
In SD 605-332-6689
Fax 605-332-6818

Smart Card

For group providers, hospitals, HMO's, group practices.
Plastic, wallet size card with integrated computer microchip; lists medical problems in a 62-item profile, including medications and interactions, insurance information, personal information, person to notify
Available from:
Smart Card Systems
15911 Forsythia Cir. (APD)
Del Ray Beach, FL 33484
407-495-2590
Fax 407-243-8740

SmartCare™

Card listed medical information, allergies, emergency phone numbers; insurance
Available from:
SmartPractice™
3400 E. McDowell (APD)
Phoenix, AZ 85008-7899
800-522-0800
Fax 800-522-8329

SportID

Rip-proof, weather proof decal and label for outside of helmet and bicycle frame; room for name, address, phone,

Allergy Products Directory
Copyrighted. Reproduction Prohibited by Law. 1259 El Camino #254, Menlo Park, CA 94025

Asthma Resources Directory
Preparing for Emergencies

emergency contact, insurance information, allergies, other medical information
Availble from
CycleAware, Inc.
655 Skyway (APD)
San Carlos, CA 94070
415-508-0599

PREPARE FOR TRAVEL EMERGENCIES

Travelers Health Hotline
CDC Voice Information System
404-332-4555
404-332-4559
24-hour information line for health advisories, vaccination recommendations, food and water safety; needs a touch-tone phone

Corporate Membership Program for Emergencies
Travelers and expatriates subscribe to service. If a health problem arises, there is a 24-hour help desk staffed by registered nurses with emergency room experience and computer-based triage system. Nurse assesses situation and refers to most appropriate, English-speaking doctor, clinic or hospital. If after hours, and emergency or urgent care is needed, Global calls to make arrangements.
Available from:
Global Emergency Medical Services
2001 Westside Dr. #120
Alpharetta, GA 30201
800-860-1111

Dept. of State Citizens Emergency Center
202-647-5225
Works with embassies to keep families informed if you are hospitalized overseas; refers to emergency medical transport companies; 8:15 am to 10:00 pm EST M-F, 9:00 am to 3:00 pm EST Sat. For

afterhours emergency contact: 202-634-3600 and ask for the duty officer of the Citizens Emergency Center

Immunization Alert!
Database of health information for travelers internationally
Available from
Immunization Alert!
PO Box 406 (APD)
Storrs, CT 06268
203-487-0002

TRAVAX
Subscription computer database of travel health information for 229 countries includes health and safety information. Itinerary check: enter countries for specific recommendations for immunizations, travel advisories. Appropriate for hospitals, clinics, corporate health departments, military
Available from:
Shoreland Medical Marketing, Inc.
10625 W. North Ave. #209 (APD)
Milwaukee, WI 53226
PO Box 13795 (APD)
Milwauakee, WI 53213-0795
414-774-4600

Traveller Clinical Record
Folder with personal information, medications, alert for allergies, electrocardiogram, schedule of dosages for hyposensitization
Available from:
Int'l Assn. for Medical Assistance to Travellers/(IAMAT)
736 Center St. (APD)
Lewiston, NY 14092
716-754-4883
and
40 Regal Rd. (APD)
Guelph, ON N1K 1B5
Canada
and
188 Nicklin Rd. (APD)
Guelph, ON N1H 7L5
Canada
and:

121

Asthma Resources Directory

Preparing for Emergencies

Int'l Assn. for Medical Assistance
to Travellers/(IAMAT)
1287 St. Clair Ave. W. (APD)
Toronto, ON M6E 1B8
Canada
and
575 Bourke St. 12 Flr. (APD)
Melbourne 3000
Australia
and
57 Voirets (APD)
1212 Grand-Lancy, Geneva
Switzerland
and:
Int'l Assn. for Medical Assistance
to Travellers/(IAMAT)
PO Box 5049 (APD)
Christchurch 5

New Zealand

U.S.Public Health

Travel advisor gives specific
information
Chicago: 312-894-2960; 12:00 pm to
8:00 pm
Honolulu: 808-541-2552; 6:00 am to
3:00 pm
Los Angeles: 310-215-2365 8:00 am to
5:00 pm
Miami: 305-526-2910; 8:00 am to 5:00
pm
New York: 718-553-1685; 8:00 am to
10:00 pm
San Francisco: 415-876-2872; 8:00 am
to 4:30 pm

SUPPORT AND INFORMATION PROGRAMS

PROGRAMS FOR INDIVIDUALS WITH ASTHMA AND FAMILIES

"Aerosolized Medication"

Demonstration of equipment for asthma treatment by Mark Windt, MD
Available from:
Asthma Outreach Library
37 Pillsbury Rd. (APD)
Sandown, NH 03873
603-329-5301

"Asthma Medications"

Given by Frank Lukosius
Available from:
Asthma Outreach Library
37 Pillsbury Rd. (APD)
Sandown, NH 03873
603-329-5301

"Asthma: What You Need to Know"

Basic asthma information video for families, schools, or doctor's offices
Available from:
Allergy & Asthma Network/
Mothers of Asthmatics, Inc.
3554 Chain Bridge Rd. Ste 200 (APD)
Fairfax, VA 22030-2709
Orders 800-878-4403
703-385-4403
Fax 703-352-4354
and:
Asthma & Allergy Foundation of America
1125 15th St. N.W. #502 (APD)
Washington, DC 20005
202-466-7643
Fax 202-466-8940

"Essence of Life"

Asthma
Available from:
Glaxo, Inc.
5 Moore Dr. (APD)
Research Triangle Park, NC 27709

919-248-2100
Fax 919-248-2381

"Guidelines from NIH"

Albert Sheffer, MD discusses
Available from:
Asthma Outreach Library
37 Pillsbury Rd. (APD)
Sandown, NH 03873
603-329-5301

"Parent's Perspective of Asthma"

Nancy Sander
Describes concrns of parents with asthmatic children; impact on family life; ways that parents can participate in management of disease; self-management techniques for children
Available from:
American Assn. for Respiratory Care
11030 Ables Ln. (APD)
Dallas, TX 75229-4593
214-243-2272
Fax 214-484-2720

"Wheezers Anonymous"

Video tape for an adult self-management program to recognize triggers that help avoid asthma attacks; includes "Wheezers Anonymous Guidebook"
Available from:
Pulmonary Paper, The
PO Box 877 (APD)
Ormand Beach, FL 32175
800-950-3698
904-673-7501
Fax 904-673-5044

Asthma Resources Directory
Support and Information Programs

PROGRAMS FOR CHILDREN WITH ASTHMA

"Asthma Super Stars"
Video tells children that they can manage asthma
Available from:
Asthma & Allergy Foundation of America
1125 15th St. N.W. #502 (APD)
Washington, DC 20005
202-466-7643
Fax 202-466-8940

"Children's Relaxation Tape"
Available from:
Asthma Outreach Library
37 Pillsbury Rd. (APD)
Sandown, NH 03873
603-329-5301

"Free to Breathe: Inhaler Use for Children with Asthma"
Teaches children to use inhalers; encourages them to talk about their thoughts and choices
Available from:
Allergy & Asthma Network/
Mothers of Asthmatics, Inc.
3554 Chain Bridge Rd. Ste 200 (APD)
Fairfax, VA 22030-2709
Orders 800-878-4403
703-385-4403
Fax 703-352-4354

"I'm A Meter Reader"
Nancy Sander
Video in English or Spanish; book available in English or Spanish; introduces children to peak flow meters
Available from:
Allen & Hanburys™
Div. of Glaxo, Inc.
5 Moore Dr. (APD)
Research Triangle Park, NC 27709
919-248-2100
Medical services 919-248-2100
and:
Allergy & Asthma Network/

Mothers of Asthmatics, Inc.
3554 Chain Bridge Rd. Ste 200 (APD)
Fairfax, VA 22030-2709
Orders 800-878-4403
703-385-4403
Fax 703-352-4354
and:
Asthma Outreach Library
37 Pillsbury Rd. (APD)
Sandown, NH 03873
603-329-5301

"So You Have Asthma, Too!"
Nancy Sander
Video in English or Spanish; book available in English or Spanish; for young children
Available from:
Allen & Hanburys™
Div. of Glaxo, Inc.
5 Moore Dr. (APD)
Research Triangle Park, NC 27709
919-248-2100
Medical services 919-248-2100
and:
Allergy & Asthma Network/
Mothers of Asthmatics, Inc.
3554 Chain Bridge Rd. Ste 200 (APD)
Fairfax, VA 22030-2709
Orders 800-878-4403
703-385-4403
Fax 703-352-4354
and:
Asthma Outreach Library
37 Pillsbury Rd. (APD)
Sandown, NH 03873
603-329-5301

"Special Place, A"
For children
Available from:
Lordawn Enterprises
3332 Yonge St. (APD)
PO Box 94014 (APD)
Toronto, ON M4N 3R1
Canada

Asthma Resources Directory
Support and Information Programs

"Wheeze World"

In a spoof for children on "Wayne's World," Zeke and Reggie talk about fixing asthma
Available from:
Allergy & Asthma Network/
Mothers of Asthmatics, Inc.
3554 Chain Bridge Rd. Ste 200 (APD)
Fairfax, VA 22030-2709
Orders 800-878-4403
703-385-4403
Fax 703-352-4354

PROGRAMS IN SPANISH FOR CHILDREN WITH ASTHMA

"I'm A Meter Reader"
Nancy Sander
Video; book available; introduces children to peak flow meters
Available from:
Allen & Hanburys™
Div. of Glaxo, Inc.
5 Moore Dr. (APD)
Research Triangle Park, NC 27709
919-248-2100
Medical services 919-248-2100
and:
Allergy & Asthma Network/
Mothers of Asthmatics, Inc.
3554 Chain Bridge Rd. Ste 200 (APD)
Fairfax, VA 22030-2709
Orders 800-878-4403
703-385-4403
Fax 703-352-4354
and:
Asthma Outreach Library
37 Pillsbury Rd. (APD)
Sandown, NH 03873
603-329-5301

"So You Have Asthma, Too!"
Nancy Sander
Video; book available; for young children
Available from:
Allen & Hanburys™
Div. of Glaxo, Inc.

5 Moore Dr. (APD)
Research Triangle Park, NC 27709
919-248-2100
Medical services 919-248-2100
and:
Allergy & Asthma Network/
Mothers of Asthmatics, Inc.
3554 Chain Bridge Rd. Ste 200 (APD)
Fairfax, VA 22030-2709
Orders 800-878-4403
703-385-4403
Fax 703-352-4354
and:
Asthma Outreach Library
37 Pillsbury Rd. (APD)
Sandown, NH 03873
603-329-5301

PROGRAMS FOR TEENS WITH ASTHMA

"Time Out"
For teens
Available from:
Lordawn Enterprises??
3332 Yonge St. (APD)
PO Box 94014 (APD)
Toronto, ON M4N 3R1
Canada

ASTHMA EXERCISE PROGRAMS

"Aerobics for Asthmatics"
Nancy Hogshead, three-time gold medal winner at the 1984 Olylmpics, leads an aerobics class
Available from:
Allergy & Asthma Network/
Mothers of Asthmatics, Inc.
3554 Chain Bridge Rd. Ste 200 (APD)
Fairfax, VA 22030-2709
Orders 800-878-4403
703-385-4403
Fax 703-352-4354

"Chairobics Video Tape"
A program complete with education and exercise for use at home

125

Asthma Resources Directory
Support and Information Programs

Available from:
Pulmonary Paper, The
PO Box 877 (APD)
Ormand Beach, FL 32175
800-950-3698
904-673-7501
Fax 904-673-5044

"Take a Deep Breath with Terry Bradshaw"
Exercise for pulmonary patients led by Terry Bradshaw
Available from
The Pulmonary Rehabilitation Ctr. at Schumpert Medical Ctr.
One St. Mary Pl. (APD)
Shreveport, LA 71101

ASTHMA PROGRAMS FOR SCHOOLS OR COMMUNITY

"Managing Asthma in School: An Action Plan"
Basics of asthma; video shows school nurses, parents, and doctors how to work as a team
Available from:
Asthma & Allergy Foundation of America
1125 15th St. N.W. #502 (APD)
Washington, DC 20005
202-466-7643
Fax 202-466-8940

ASTHMA PROGRAMS FOR PROFESSIONALS

"Asthma and Allergy Support Groups: The Clinician's Role"
Available from:
Asthma & Allergy Foundation of America
1125 15th St. N.W. #502 (APD)
Washington, DC 20005
202-466-7643
Fax 202-466-8940

"New Concepts in Asthma Therapy"
Paul C. Stillwell, MD
Discusses medication delivery devices, anticholinergics, cromolyn use, steroid controversies, emergency room procedures, outpatient therapy
Available from:
American Assn. for Respiratory Care
11030 Ables Ln. (APD)
Dallas, TX 75229-4593
214-243-2272
Fax 214-484-2720

"New Treatments for Asthma"
Roger Bone, MD
For professionals. Dr. Bone discusses patient education and self-management programs using a peak flow meter; explains "step-care" treatment
Available from:
American Assn. for Respiratory Care
11030 Ables Ln. (APD)
Dallas, TX 75229-4593
214-243-2272
Fax 214-484-2720

Allergy Products Directory
Copyrighted. Reproduction Prohibited by Law. 1259 El Camino #254, Menlo Park, CA 94025

Asthma Resources Directory

Newsletters

NEWSLETTERS AND DIRECTORIES

FOR PATIENTS AND THEIR FAMILIES

"AAAR Times"
Available from:
American Assn. for Respiratory Care
11030 Ables Ln. (APD)
Dallas, TX 75229-4593
214-243-2272
Fax 214-484-2720

"Advance"
Available from:
Asthma & Allergy Foundation of America
1125 15th St. N.W. #502 (APD)
Washington, DC 20005
202-466-7643
Fax 202-466-8940

"Air Currents"
Available from:
Allen & Hanburys™
Div. of Glaxo, Inc.
5 Moore Dr. (APD)
Research Triangle Park, NC 27709
919-248-2100
Medical services 919-248-2100

"Airways"
Quarterly
Available from:
Allergy & Asthma Center
2233-F Willamette (APD)
Eugene, OR 97401
503-485-0316

"Allergy Answers"
Available from:
Demos Publications
156 Fifth Ave. Ste 1018 (APD)
New York, NY 10010
212-255-8768

"Allergy Forum™"
(available through doctor's office)

"American Lung Association, Bulletin"
Available from:
American Lung Assn.
800-LUNG-USA (5864-872)
Refers to local ALA for information

"Asthma and Allergy Advocate"
Available from:
American Academy Allergy/Imm.
611 E. Wells St. 4th Flr. (APD)
Milwaukee, WI 53202-3816
800-822-ASMA (2762)
414-272-6071
Fax 414-276-3349

"Asthma Update"
Available from:
Asthma Update
123 Monticello Ave. (APD)
Annapolis, MD 21401
410-267-0309

"Healthlines"
(for and by teens)
Available from:
Asthma & Allergy Foundation of America
1125 15th St. N.W. #502 (APD)
Washington, DC 20005
202-466-7643
Fax 202-466-8940

"LungLine Letter"
Available from:
National Jewish Center for Immunology
and Respiratory Medicine
1400 Jackson at ColFax (APD)
Denver, CO 80206-2762
800-222-LUNG (5864)
In CO 303-355-LUNG (5864)
303-398-1907

"New Directions"
For donors
Available from:

127

Asthma Resources Directory

Newsletters

National Jewish Center for
Immunology
and Respiratory Medicine
1400 Jackson at ColFax (APD)
Denver, CO 80206-2762
800-222-LUNG (5864)
In CO 303-355-LUNG (5864)
303-398-1907

"MA Report"
Available from:
Allergy & Asthma Network/
Mothers of Asthmatics, Inc.
3554 Chain Bridge Rd. Ste 200 (APD)
Fairfax, VA 22030-2709
Orders 800-878-4403
703-385-4403
Fax 703-352-4354

FOR PROFESSIONALS IN THE FIELD

"Medical/Scientific UPDATE"
Available from:
National Jewish Center for
Immunology
and Respiratory Medicine
1400 Jackson at ColFax (APD)
Denver, CO 80206-2762
800-222-LUNG (5864)
In CO 303-355-LUNG (5864)
303-398-1907

IN OTHER COUNTRIES

"Allergy Asthma Quarterly"
Available from:
Allergy/Asthma Information Assn.
30 Eglinton Ave. W. #750 (APD)
Mississauga, ON L5R 3E7
Canada
905-712-AAIA (2242)
Fax 905-712-2245

"Asthma Network"
Available from:
World Network of Asthma
Organizations
Canadian Secretariat

c/o Canadian Lung Assn.
1900 City Park Dr. #508 (APD)
Gloucester, ON K1J 1A3
Canada
613-747-6766
Fax 613-747-7430

"Easy Breathing"
Manitoba Lung Assn.
629 McDermot Ave. 2nd Flr. (APD)
Winnipeg, MB R3A 5P6
Canada

"Newsletter for People with Lung Problems, A"
Lung Assn. (Metro, Toronto, York
Region)
573 King St. E. Ste. 201 (APD)
Toronto, ON M5A 1M5
Canada

"Canadian Society for Immunology, Bulletin"
(for professionals in the field)
Canadian Society for Immunology
Dr. C. Ottaway
St. Michael's Univ. of Toronto
Toronto, ON M5S 1A8
Canada

OF RELATED INTEREST

"ACCH Network"
Available from:
Assn. for Care of Children's Health
7910 Woodmont Ave. #300 (APD)
Bethesda, MD 20814-3015
301-654-6549
Fax 301-986-4553

"Americans for Nonsmokers' Rights Update"
Available from:
Americans for Nonsmokers' Rights
2530 San Pablo Ave. #J (APD)
Berkeley, CA 94702
PO Box 668 (APD)
Berkeley, CA 94704
510-841-3032

Asthma Resources Directory

Newsletters

"ASH Smoking and Health Review"
Available from:
Action on Smoking and Health
2013 H St. N.W. (APD)
Washington, DC 20006
202-659-4310

"Common Sense Pest Control"
Available from:
Bio-Integral Resource Center, The
PO Box 7414 (APD)
Berkeley, CA 94707
510-524-2567
Fax 510-524-1758

"Drugs & Therapeutics"
Available from:
Drug Information Center - Mercy
Mercy Hospital of Pittsburgh
1400 Locust St. (APD)
Pittsburgh , PA 15219-5166
412-232-7903 (APD)

"HealthFacts"
Consumer-oriented, general, medical information
Available from:
Comfortably Yours
2515 E. 43rd St. (APD)
Chattanooga, TN 37422
201-368-0400

"Health Gazette: A Digest of Medical Facts and News"
Available from:
Health Gazette®
PO Box 1786 (APD)
Indiannapolis, IN 46206
317-253-7104
Fax 317-253-8582

"Helping Ourselves"
Available from:
Michigan Self-Help Clearinghouse (Regional)
106 W. Allegan #210 (APD)
Lansing, MI 48933-1706
MI 800-777-5556

Business line 517-484-7373

"Indoor Air Quality Updates"
(for Professionals)
Available from
Cutter Information Corp.
37 Broadway (APD)
Arlington, MA 02174-5539
800-964-5118
617-641-5118
Fax 800-888-1816
Fax 617-648-1950

"Lifeline"
Available from:
Celiac Sprue Assn./
United States of America
PO Box 31700 (APD)
Omaha, NE 68131-0700
402-558-0600

"Network"
(self-help clearinghouse)
Available from:
New Jersey Self-Help Clearinhouse (Regional)
St. Clares-Riverside Med. Center
Pocono Rd. (APD)
Denville, NJ 07834
NJ 800-FOR-MASH (367-6274)
201-625-9565
TDD 201-625-9053

"NSHC Newsletter"
Available from:
National Self-Help Clearinghouse
25 W. 43rd St. Rm. 620 (APD)
New York, NY 10036
212-642-2944
NY City Referrals 212-586-5770
Fax 212-719-2488

"Pediatrics for Parents"
Available from:
Pediatrics for Parents
358 Broadway #105 (APD)
Bangor, ME 04401
207-942-6212

Asthma Resources Directory

Newsletters

"Today's Medicines"
Available from:
Michigan Pharmacists Assn.
815 N. Washington Ave. (APD)
Lansing, MI 48906
517-484-1466

DIRECTORIES
IN ALLERGY AND ASTHMA

"AAA Resource Handbook"
Covers services, products, and sources of information
Available from:
AROA/Allergy Assn. Australia
PO Box 298 (APD)
Ringwood, Vic 3134
Australia

"Allergy/Asthma Finding Help"
National and international sources of written, personal, and computerized help
Available from:
Allergy Publications
PO Box 640 (APD)
Menlo Park, CA 94026
415-322-1663

"Controlling Your Environment"
Articles cover methods of environmental improvement with lists of products and where to buy them
Available from:
Allergy Publications
PO Box 640 (APD)
Menlo Park, CA 94026
415-322-1663

"Grocery Manufacturers Directory"
Phone numbers
Available from:
Food Allergy Network, The
4744 Holly Ave. (APD)
Fairfax, VA 22030-5647
703-691-3179

"Health Care Resource Directory
National sources of health care information
Available from:
Metro Publishing
5308 Elm St., Bldg C (APD)
Houston, TX 77081
800-473-5555
713-666-7841

Allergy Products Directory
Copyrighted. Reproduction Prohibited by Law. 1259 El Camino #254, Menlo Park, CA 94025

Asthma Resources Directory

Information In Print

ASTHMA INFORMATION IN PRINT

Some books may not be readily available through a bookstore, even with a special order. Try your library. Ask about an inter-library loan or write the publisher.

Some books are out of print. Used book stores may be able to list the book you want in *A Bookman's Weekly* for a small fee. Be patient. A response can take months. Try *Guide to Out-of-Print Books*. It is a catalogue on microfiche and is available for free from UMI at PO Box 1467, Ann Arbor, MI 48106; 800-521-0600. You can most likely use your library's microfiche system to read it.

INFORMATION IN PRINT

"About Asthma"
Available from:
American Lung Assn.
800-LUNG-USA (5864-872)
Refers to local ALA for information

"Air Purifiers Part 1 Claims, Types"
Available from:
American Allergy Assn.
1259 El Camino #254 (APD)
Menlo Park, CA 94025
415-322-1663
Internet AllergyAid@aol.com

"Air Purifiers Part II Considerations, Testing, Questions"
Available from:
American Allergy Assn.
1259 El Camino #254 (APD)
Menlo Park, CA 94025
415-322-1663
Internet AllergyAid@aol.com

"All About Asthma"
William Ostrow
Vivian Ostrow
Available from:
A. Whitman, Albert & Co.
5747 W. Howard St. (APD)
Niles, IL 60648
and:
Asthma & Allergy Foundation of America

1125 15th St. N.W. #502 (APD)
Washington, DC 20005
202-466-7643
Fax 202-466-8940
and:
Asthma Outreach Library
37 Pillsbury Rd. (APD)
Sandown, NH 03873
603-329-5301

"All About Asthma"
Glennon Paul, MD
Barbara A. Fafoglia
Available from:
Asthma Outreach Library
37 Pillsbury Rd. (APD)
Sandown, NH 03873
603-329-5301
and:
Sterling Publishing Co., Inc.
387 Park Ave. S. (APD)
New York, NY 10016-8810
NY 212-532-7160
800-367-9692

"Allergy & Asthma '95"
Annually
Available from:
Healthline Publishing, Inc.
830 Menlo Ave. #100
Menlo Park, CA 94025
800-766-5566
325-6457

Asthma Resources Directory

Information In Print

"Allergy Alerts from Living with Allergies"
Available from:
American Allergy Assn.
1259 El Camino #254 (APD)
Menlo Park, CA 94025
415-322-1663
Internet AllergyAid@aol.com

"Allergy Products Directory"
Controlling Your Environment
Allergy/Asthma Finding Help
Asthma Resources Directory
Food Allergy Resources
Available from:
Allergy Publications
1259 El Camino #254 (APD)
Menlo Park, CA 94025
415-322-1663

"Americans with Disabilities Act"
Available from:
Asthma & Allergy Foundation of America
1125 15th St. N.W. #502 (APD)
Washington, DC 20005
202-466-7643
Fax 202-466-8940

"An Introduction to Your Child Who Has Asthma"
W. Linaweaver, Jr., MD, et. al.
Available from:
Medic Publishing
PO Box 89 (APD)
Redmond, CA 98073

"As You Live...And Breathe"
Available from:
American Lung Assn.
800-LUNG-USA (5864-872)
Refers to local ALA for information

"Asthma Alert for School Administrators"
Available from:
American Lung Assn.
800-LUNG-USA (5864-872)
Refers to local ALA for information

"Asthma Alert for School Nurses"
ALA/Middlesex County
5 Mountain Rd. (APD)
PO Box 265 (APD)
Burlington, MA 01803-0465
617-272-2866

"Asthma Alert for Teachers"
Available from:
American Lung Assn.
800-LUNG-USA (5864-872)
Refers to local ALA for information

"Asthma and Allergic Diseases"
J. D. Wilson
Available from:
Charles B. Stack, Inc.
6900 Grove Rd. (APD)
Thorofare, NJ 08036
800-257-8290
NJ 609-848-1000

"Asthma and Allergy Medicines: Side Effects"
Available from:
Asthma & Allergy Foundation of America
1125 15th St. N.W. #502 (APD)
Washington, DC 20005
202-466-7643
Fax 202-466-8940

"Asthma and Exercise"
Nancy Hogshead
Gerald S. Couzens
Available from:
Allergy & Asthma Network/
Mothers of Asthmatics, Inc.
3554 Chain Bridge Rd. Ste 200 (APD)
Fairfax, VA 22030-2709
Orders 800-878-4403
703-385-4403
Fax 703-352-4354
and:
Allergy Solutions
4909 W. Park Blvd. #169 (APD)
Plano, TX 75093
800-380-SNEEZ (7633)
214-612-4188
Fax 214-985-5573

132

Allergy Products Directory
Copyrighted. Reproduction Prohibited by Law. 1259 El Camino #254, Menlo Park, CA 94025

Asthma Resources Directory

Information In Print

and:
Asthma Outreach Library
37 Pillsbury Rd. (APD)
Sandown, NH 03873
603-329-5301
and:
Henry Holt & Co.
115 W. 18th St. (APD)
New York, NY 10011
NY 212-886-9200
800-247-3912

"Asthma and Hay Fever"
Alan Knight
Available from:
Arco Publishing, Inc.
219 Park Ave. S. (APD)
New York, NY 10003-1601

"Asthma and Hay Fever"
Oscar Swineford, Jr.
Available from:
Charles C Thomas, Publisher
2600 S. First St. (APD)
Springfield, IL 62794-9265

"Asthma Basics"
Available from:
Asthma & Allergy Foundation of
America
1125 15th St. N.W. #502 (APD)
Washington, DC 20005
202-466-7643
Fax 202-466-8940

"Asthma Facts"
Available from:
American Lung Assn.
800-LUNG-USA (5864-872)
Refers to local ALA for information

"Asthma Handbook"
Stuart H. Young, MD
Susan A. Shulman
Martin D. Shulman, PhD
Available from:
American Lung Assn.
800-LUNG-USA (5864-872)
Refers to local ALA for information

and:
Bantam Books, Inc.
Div. of Bantam/Doubleday/Dell Pub.
666 Fifth Ave. (APD)
New York, NY 10103

"Asthma Handbook, The"
Available from:
American Lung Assn.
800-LUNG-USA (5864-872)
Refers to local ALA for information

"Asthma Handbook, The: A Complete Guide for Patients and Their Families"
Stuart H. Young
Susan A. Schulman
Martin D. Schulman
Available from:
Bantam Books, Inc.
Div. of Bantam/Doubleday/Dell Pub.
666 Fifth Ave. (APD)
New York, NY 10103

"Asthma in the School: Improving Control with Peak Flow Monitoring"
Guillermo Mendoza, MD
Mary Garcia, RN, MN
Mary Collins, MA
Available from:
Allen & Hanburys™
Div. of Glaxo, Inc.
5 Moore Dr. (APD)
Research Triangle Park, NC 27709
919-248-2100
Medical services 919-248-2100
and:
Allergy & Asthma Network/
Mothers of Asthmatics, Inc.
3554 Chain Bridge Rd. Ste 200 (APD)
Fairfax, VA 22030-2709
Orders 800-878-4403
703-385-4403
Fax 703-352-4354
and:
Asthma & Allergy Foundation of
America
1125 15th St. N.W. #502 (APD)
Washington, DC 20005

Asthma Resources Directory

Information In Print

202-466-7643
Fax 202-466-8940
and:
Asthma Outreach Library
37 Pillsbury Rd. (APD)
Sandown, NH 03873
603-329-5301

"Asthma in the Workplace"
Available from:
Asthma & Allergy Foundation of
America
1125 15th St. N.W. #502 (APD)
Washington, DC 20005
202-466-7643
Fax 202-466-8940

"Asthma Medication"
Joann Blessing-Moore, MD
Available from:
American Allergy Assn.
1259 El Camino #254 (APD)
Menlo Park, CA 94025
415-322-1663
Internet AllergyAid@aol.com

"Asthma Organizer"
Nancy Sander
Debra Scherrer
Martha White, MD
Available from:
Allergy & Asthma Network/
Mothers of Asthmatics, Inc.
3554 Chain Bridge Rd. Ste 200 (APD)
Fairfax, VA 22030-2709
Orders 800-878-4403
703-385-4403
Fax 703-352-4354

"Asthma Reading and Resource List"
Available from:
National Heart, Lung/Blood Inst.
NIH Asthma Project
Bldg. 31, Rm. 4A-21
9000 Rockville Pike (APD)
Bethesda, MD 20892-0001
301-496-4236
301-496-2411

"Asthma Self-Care Book"
Geri Harrington
Available from:
Allergy Solutions
4909 W. Park Blvd. #169 (APD)
Plano, TX 75093
800-380-SNEEZ (7633)
214-612-4188
Fax 214-985-5573
and:
Pulmonary Paper, The
PO Box 877 (APD)
Ormand Beach, FL 32175
800-950-3698
904-673-7501
Fax 904-673-5044

"Asthma Self-Help Book: How to Live a Normal Life in Spite of Your Condition"
Paul J. Hannaway, MD
Available from:
Allergy Asthma Technology
4151 N. Kedzie (APD)
PO Box 18398 (APD)
Chicago, IL 60618
800-621-5545
312-465-8020
Fax 312-465-7619
and:
Allergy Solutions
4909 W. Park Blvd. #169 (APD)
Plano, TX 75093
800-380-SNEEZ (7633)
214-612-4188
Fax 214-985-5573
and:
Prima Publishing Co.
PO Box 1260 (APD)
Rocklin, CA 95677-1260
916-786-0426

"Asthma Storm"
Barbara Westmoreland, RN
Available from
Lane Publishers

"Asthma"
G. Clark
Available from:

Asthma Resources Directory

Information In Print

Year Book Medical Publications
Subs. of Times Mirror Co.
200 N. La Salle St. (APD)
Chicago, IL 60601
312-726-9746
800-622-5410

"Asthma"
Available from:
National Institute of Allergy
& Infectious Diseases
NIH - Public Health Services
Bldg. 31 Rm. 72-32 (APD)
Public Health Services
9000 Rockville Pike
Bethesda, MD 20892-0001
301-496-5717
301-496-4000

"Asthma. . .At My Age?"
Available from:
American Lung Assn.
800-LUNG-USA (5864-872)
Refers to local ALA for information

"Asthma: Airway Involvement"
Available from:
American Allergy Assn.
1259 El Camino #254 (APD)
Menlo Park, CA 94025
415-322-1663
Internet AllergyAid@aol.com

"Asthma: Description & Diagnosis"
HHS
Available from:
American Allergy Assn.
1259 El Camino #254 (APD)
Menlo Park, CA 94025
415-322-1663
Internet AllergyAid@aol.com

"Asthma: Fact & Fiction"
Linda Alpert, RN, BSN
Available from:
Asthma Foundation of Southern
Arizona
National Foundation for Asthma
PO Box 30069 (APD)

Tucson, AZ 85751-0069
520-323-6046

"Asthma: Other Physical Effects"
Available from:
American Allergy Assn.
1259 El Camino #254 (APD)
Menlo Park, CA 94025
415-322-1663
Internet AllergyAid@aol.com

"Asthma: Stop Suffering and Start Living"
M. Eric Gershwin, MD
Edwin L. Klingelhofer, PhD
Available from:
Addison-Wesley Publishing Co.
Medical\Nursing Division
1 Jacob Way (APD)
Reading, MA 01867
617-944-3700
800-447-2227
and:
Allergy Solutions
4909 W. Park Blvd. #169 (APD)
Plano, TX 75093
800-380-SNEEZ (7633)
214-612-4188
Fax 214-985-5573
and:
Asthma Outreach Library
37 Pillsbury Rd. (APD)
Sandown, NH 03873
603-329-5301
and:
Pulmonary Paper, The
PO Box 877 (APD)
Ormand Beach, FL 32175
800-950-3698
904-673-7501
Fax 904-673-5044

"Asthma: The Complete Guide to Self-Management of Asthma & Allergies for Patients & Their Families"
Allan M. Weinstein, MD
Available from:
Allergy & Asthma Network/
Mothers of Asthmatics, Inc.

Asthma Resources Directory

Information In Print

3554 Chain Bridge Rd. Ste 200 (APD)
Fairfax, VA 22030-2709
Orders 800-878-4403
703-385-4403
Fax 703-352-4354
and:
Allergy Solutions
4909 W. Park Blvd. #169 (APD)
Plano, TX 75093
800-380-SNEEZ (7633)
214-612-4188
Fax 214-985-5573
and:
Asthma & Allergy Foundation of
America
1125 15th St. N.W. #502 (APD)
Washington, DC 20005
202-466-7643
Fax 202-466-8940
and:
Asthma Outreach Library
37 Pillsbury Rd. (APD)
Sandown, NH 03873
603-329-5301
and:
McGraw-Hill Publishing Co.
1221 Avenue of the Americas (APD)
New York, NY 10020
in NY 212-512-2000
800-722-4726

"Asthma: The Facts"
Donald J. Lane
Anthony Storr
Available from:
Oxford University Press
200 Madison Ave. (APD)
New York, NY 10016
800-334-4249
212-679-7300
Orders 800-451-7556

"Being Close"
Available from:
National Jewish Center for
Immunology
and Respiratory Medicine
1400 Jackson at ColFax (APD)
Denver, CO 80206-2762
800-222-LUNG (5864)

In CO 303-355-LUNG (5864)
303-398-1907

"Best Guide to Allergies, The"
A. Giannini, MD, et. al.
Available from:
Consumers Union
256 Washington St. (APD)
Mt. Vernon, NY 10553

"Best of the MA Report"
Articles from past issues of
newsletter
Available from:
Allergy & Asthma Network/
Mothers of Asthmatics, Inc.
3554 Chain Bridge Rd. Ste 200 (APD)
Fairfax, VA 22030-2709
Orders 800-878-4403
703-385-4403
Fax 703-352-4354

"Breathe Easy: An Asthmatic's Guide to Clean Air"
Stanley Reichman
Thomas Y. Crowell Co.

"Breathing Easier"
For availability call your local
VitalAire branch
Available from:
Associated Respiratory Services
15363 11 Ave. (APD)
Edmonton, AB T5M 3X4
Canada

"Breathing Easy with Day Care"
Available from:
Allergy & Asthma Network/
Mothers of Asthmatics, Inc.
3554 Chain Bridge Rd. Ste 200 (APD)
Fairfax, VA 22030-2709
Orders 800-878-4403
703-385-4403
Fax 703-352-4354

"Breathing Easy: A Handbook for Asthmatics"
Genell Sabak-Sharpe
Available from:

Asthma Resources Directory

Doubleday & Co.
Div. of Bantam Doubleday Dell
666 Fifth Ave.
New York, NY 10103
800-223-6834 Ext. 479
NY 212-765-6500

"Breathing Easy: A Parent' Guide to Dealing with Your Child's Asthma"
Maryann Stevens
Available from:
Prentice Hall
Div. of Simon & Schuster, Inc.
15 Columbus Cir. (APD)
New York, NY 10023
800-922-0579
212-373-8500

"Breathing Exercises for Asthma"
Karen R. Butts
Available from:
Charles C Thomas, Publisher
2600 S. First St. (APD)
Springfield, IL 62794-9265

"Breathing Exercises for Asthma"
CKRB Publishers
Karen R. Butts

"Canadian Allergy & Asthma Handbook"
Barry Zimmerman, MD
Milton Gold, MD
Sasson Lavi, MD
Stephen Feanny, MD
Available from:
Random House, Inc.
201 E. 50th St. 31st Flr. (APD)
New York, NY 10022
212-751-2600
Orders 800-733-3000
Inquiries 800-726-0600

"Child with Asthma, The"
Rosemary Dinnage
Stan Gooch
Available from:
NFER-Nelson
Windsor, Berkshire

England

"Childhood Asthma: A Guide for Parents"
P.A. Eggleston, MD
Available from:
Asthma & Allergy Foundation of America
1125 15th St. N.W. #502 (APD)
Washington, DC 20005
202-466-7643
Fax 202-466-8940

"Childhood Asthma: A Matter of Control"
Available from:
American Lung Assn.
800-LUNG-USA (5864-872)
Refers to local ALA for information

"Children with Asthma: A Manual for Parents"
Thomas F. Plaut, MD
Available from:
Allergy Asthma Technology
4151 N. Kedzie (APD)
PO Box 18398 (APD)
Chicago, IL 60618
800-621-5545
312-465-8020
Fax 312-465-7619
and:
Allergy Clean Environments
501 Station Ave. (APD)
Haddon Heights, NJ 08035
800-882-4110
In NJ 609-546-1101
Fax 609-546-1466
URL:
http:\\WWW.infomall.com\allergy.html
and:
Asthma & Allergy Foundation of America
1125 15th St. N.W. #502 (APD)
Washington, DC 20005
202-466-7643
Fax 202-466-8940
and:
Asthma Outreach Library
37 Pillsbury Rd. (APD)

137

Asthma Resources Directory

Information In Print

Sandown, NH 03873
603-329-5301
and:
Pedipress, Inc.
125 Red Gate Lane (APD)
Amherst, MA 01002

Clean Air Booklets
"Air Pollution in Your Home"
"Don't You Dare Breathe that Air"
"Get a Check-up for Your Car!" (in
Spanish also)
"Home Indoor Air Quality Checklist"
(in Spanish also)
"Indoor Air Pollution in the Office"
"Office Indoor Air Quality Checklist"
Available from:
American Lung Assn.
800-LUNG-USA (5864-872)
Refers to local ALA for information

"Complete Book of Children's Allergies, The"
Robert B. Feldman
David Carroll
Available from:
Delta Delacorte
Div. of Bantam Doubleday Dell
666th Ave. (APD)
New York, NY 10103
800-221-4676
212-765-6500
and:
Warner Books, Inc.
1271 Ave. of the Americas (APD)
New York, NY 10020
212-522-7200

"Conquering Asthma: An Illustrated Guide to Self Care"
Michael T. Newhouse, MD
Peter J. Barnes, MD
Available from:
Decker Periodicals, Inc.
1 James St. (APD)
PO Box 620 LCD1 (APD)
Hamilton, ON L8N 3K7
Canada

"Consumer Guide for Room Air Cleaners"
Available from:
Assn. of Home Appliance
Manufacturers
AHAM
20 N. Wacker Dr. (APD)
Chicago, IL 60606
312-984-5800

"Consumer Update on Asthma"
Nancy Sander
Available from:
Allergy & Asthma Network/
Mothers of Asthmatics, Inc.
3554 Chain Bridge Rd. Ste 200 (APD)
Fairfax, VA 22030-2709
Orders 800-878-4403
703-385-4403
Fax 703-352-4354

"Controlling Asthma"
Available from:
American Lung Assn.
800-LUNG-USA (5864-872)
Refers to local ALA for information

"Directions for Use of Ana-Kit®/Ana-Guard™ Epinephrine Syringe"
Available from:
Miles Inc. Pharmaceutical Div.
Miles Allergy Products
(Hollister-Stier)
PO Box 3145 (APD)
3525 N. Regal (APD)
Spokane, WA 99220-3145
800-992-1120
509-489-5656

"Down with the Dust Mite"
Available from:
American Allergy Assn.
1259 El Camino #254 (APD)
Menlo Park, CA 94025
415-322-1663
Internet AllergyAid@aol.com

"Drug Allergy"
Available from:

Asthma Resources Directory

Information In Print

National Institute of Allergy
& Infectious Diseases
NIH - Public Health Services
Bldg. 31 Rm. 72-32 (APD)
Public Health Services
9000 Rockville Pike
Bethesda, MD 20892-0001
301-496-5717
301-496-4000

"Dust 'n' Stuff"
Linda Alpert, RN, BSN
Available from:
Asthma Foundation of Southern
Arizona
National Foundation for Asthma
PO Box 30069 (APD)
Tucson, AZ 85751-0069
520-323-6046

"Dust Allergy"
Available from:
National Institute of Allergy
& Infectious Diseases
NIH - Public Health Services
Bldg. 31 Rm. 72-32 (APD)
Public Health Services
9000 Rockville Pike
Bethesda, MD 20892-0001
301-496-5717
301-496-4000

"Electronic Air Cleaners and HEPA Filters, Ion Machines, Portable Air Cleaners"
J. Gordon King
Available from:
American Allergy Assn.
1259 El Camino #254 (APD)
Menlo Park, CA 94025
415-322-1663
Internet AllergyAid@aol.com

"Electronic Air Cleaners, HEPA Filters"
J. Gordon King
Available from:
American Allergy Assn.
1259 El Camino #254 (APD)
Menlo Park, CA 94025

415-322-1663
Internet AllergyAid@aol.com

"Empty Your Bucket: Practical Steps to Overcome Allergy and Allergic Asthma"
Stephen H. Astor, MD
Available from:
Priorities®
70 Walnut St. (APD)
Wellesley, MA 02181
800-553-5398
and:
Two A's Industries, Inc.
285 South Dr. (APD)
Mountain View, CA 94040-4318
415-968-3111

"Ensuring Clean Indoor Air"
Judy Lee Bachman, PhD
Available from:
Health Services Consultants
2670 Del Mar Heights Rd. #194 (APD)
Del Mar, CA 92014

"Environmental Allergens Part 1 House Dust, Control of House Dust"
Available from:
American Allergy Assn.
1259 El Camino #254 (APD)
Menlo Park, CA 94025
415-322-1663
Internet AllergyAid@aol.com

"Environmental Allergens Part 2 Dog and Cat Sensititivity"
Available from:
American Allergy Assn.
1259 El Camino #254 (APD)
Menlo Park, CA 94025
415-322-1663
Internet AllergyAid@aol.com

"Environmental Allergens Part 3 Pollen Allergy, Mold Spores, Other"
Available from:
American Allergy Assn.
1259 El Camino #254 (APD)

Asthma Resources Directory

Information In Print

Menlo Park, CA 94025
415-322-1663
Internet AllergyAid@aol.com

"Essential Asthma Book, The: A Manual for Asthmatics of all Ages"
Francois Haas, MD
Sheila Sperber Haas, MD
Available from:
Allergy Solutions
4909 W. Park Blvd. #169 (APD)
Plano, TX 75093
800-380-SNEEZ (7633)
214-612-4188
Fax 214-985-5573
and:
Asthma Outreach Library
37 Pillsbury Rd. (APD)
Sandown, NH 03873
603-329-5301
and:
Charles Scribner's Sons
Front & Brown Sts. (APD)
Riverside, NJ 08075

"Exercise and Allergy"
Donald L. Unger, MD
Available from:
American Allergy Assn.
1259 El Camino #254 (APD)
Menlo Park, CA 94025
415-322-1663
Internet AllergyAid@aol.com

"Exercise and Asthma"
Available from:
Asthma & Allergy Foundation of America
1125 15th St. N.W. #502 (APD)
Washington, DC 20005
202-466-7643
Fax 202-466-8940

"Exercise-Induced Asthma"
Joann Blessing-Moore, MD
Available from:
American Allergy Assn.
1259 El Camino #254 (APD)
Menlo Park, CA 94025

415-322-1663
Internet AllergyAid@aol.com

"Facts About...Asthma, The"
Available from:
American Lung Assn.
800-LUNG-USA (5864-872)
Refers to local ALA for information

"For the Teacher of the Child with Asthma"
Available from:
American Lung Assn.
800-LUNG-USA (5864-872)
Refers to local ALA for information

"Four Signs of Asthma Trouble, The"
(Free with long SASE)
Thomas F. Plaut, MD
Available from:
Pedipress, Inc.
125 Red Gate Lane (APD)
Amherst, MA 01002

"Guide to Seasonal Allergens"
Available from:
Schering Corp.
2000 Galloping Hill Rd. (APD)
Kenilworth, NJ 07033
201-558-4000

"Guidelines for the Diagnosis and Management of Asthma"
Available from:
Asthma Information Center
Nat'l Heart, Lung & Blood Inst.
4733 Bethesda Ave. #530 (APD)
Bethedsda, MD 20814
301-951-3260
and:
National Institutes of Health
9000 Rockville Pike (APD)
Bethesda, MD 20892-0001
301-496-4000
Fax 301-496-2443

"Healthy Breathing"
Available from:
National Jewish Center for Immunology

Asthma Resources Directory

Information In Print

and Respiratory Medicine
1400 Jackson at ColFax (APD)
Denver, CO 80206-2762
800-222-LUNG (5864)
In CO 303-355-LUNG (5864)
303-398-1907

"Hidden Asthma...and Other Non-classical Formats"
H. Chai, MD
Available from:
American Allergy Assn.
1259 El Camino #254 (APD)
Menlo Park, CA 94025
415-322-1663
Internet AllergyAid@aol.com

"Hints for Control of the Home Environment for the Allergic Person"
Available from:
American Lung Assn.
800-LUNG-USA (5864-872)
Refers to local ALA for information

"Holiday Allergies: 'Tis the Season!"
Available from:
Asthma & Allergy Foundation of America
1125 15th St. N.W. #502 (APD)
Washington, DC 20005
202-466-7643
Fax 202-466-8940

"How to Create a Clean Room"
Available from:
Summit Hill Laboratories
Ship to 429 Highway 36 (APD)
Mail to PO Box 535 (APD)
Navesink, NJ 07752
800-922-0722
201-291-3600

"How to Keep Your Lungs Healthy"
Available from:
American Lung Assn.
800-LUNG-USA (5864-872)
Refers to local ALA for information

"How to Use Respirators"
Available from:
Gempler's
211 Blue Mounds Rd. (APD)
PO Box 270 (APD)
Mt. Horeb, WI 53572
800-382-8473
Fax 800-551-1128

"Insect Allergy"
Available from:
National Institute of Allergy
& Infectious Diseases
NIH - Public Health Services
Bldg. 31 Rm. 72-32 (APD)
Public Health Services
9000 Rockville Pike
Bethesda, MD 20892-0001
301-496-5717
301-496-4000

"Learning to Live with Asthma"
Available from:
Boehringer Ingelheim Pharmaceuticals, Inc.
90 E. Ridge (APD)
PO Box 368 (APD)
Ridgefield, CT 06877
203-438-0311

"Living Well with Chronic Asthma, Bronchitis, and Emphysema"
Dr. M. Shayevitz
Dr. B. Shayevitz
Available from:
Consumer Reports Books
9180 LeSaint Dr. (APD)
Fairfield, OH 45014-5452
513-860-1178
Fax 513-874-1699

"Living with Allergies"
Available from:
American Allergy Assn.
1259 El Camino #254 (APD)
Menlo Park, CA 94025
415-322-1663
Internet AllergyAid@aol.com

Asthma Resources Directory

Information In Print

"Living with Asthma: A Manual for Teaching Children Self-Management of Asthma"

Thomas L. Creer
Mary Backiel
Patrick Leung
Available from:
National Heart, Lung/Blood Inst.
NIH Asthma Project
Bldg. 31, Rm. 4A-21
9000 Rockville Pike (APD)
Bethesda, MD 20892-0001
301-496-4236
301-496-2411

"Living with Your Allergies and Asthma"

Theodore Berland
Lucia Fischer-Pap
Available from:
St. Martin's Press, Inc.
175 Fifth Ave. (APD)
New York, NY 10010

"Management of Chronic Respiratory Disease"

Available from:
National Jewish Center for
Immunology
and Respiratory Medicine
1400 Jackson at ColFax (APD)
Denver, CO 80206-2762
800-222-LUNG (5864)
In CO 303-355-LUNG (5864)
303-398-1907

"Managing Childhood Asthma"

Information for parents
Available from:
Allergy & Asthma Network/
Mothers of Asthmatics, Inc.
3554 Chain Bridge Rd. Ste 200 (APD)
Fairfax, VA 22030-2709
Orders 800-878-4403
703-385-4403
Fax 703-352-4354

"Manual of Problems in Asthma, Allergy, and Related Disorders"

B. Bukstein, Editor

R. Strunk, Editor
Available from:
Little, Brown & Co.
Div. of Time, Inc.
34 Beacon St. (APD)
Boston, MA 02108
800-343-9204
MA 617-227-0730

Medical Fact Sheets

Asthma: Pregnancy, Parenting,
Early Warning Signs, Chest
Assessment, Teacher Memo. Sinusitis,
Antibiotics, Triggers, Exercise,
Nocturnal, Drugs, Over-the-Counter,
reading list, Eczema/Atopic
Dermatitis, Metered-Dose Inhalers,
Peak Flow Meter, Spirometry, Steroids,
Theophylline
Available from:
National Jewish Center for
Immunology
and Respiratory Medicine
1400 Jackson at ColFax (APD)
Denver, CO 80206-2762
800-222-LUNG (5864)
In CO 303-355-LUNG (5864)
303-398-1907

"Metered Dose Inhalers: Are You Using Yours Correctly?"

Available from:
Asthma & Allergy Foundation of
America
1125 15th St. N.W. #502 (APD)
Washington, DC 20005
202-466-7643
Fax 202-466-8940

"National Asthma Self-Education Course"

Available from:
Asthma Outreach Library
37 Pillsbury Rd. (APD)
Sandown, NH 03873
603-329-5301
and:
Asthma Today
412 State St. (APD)
Bangor, ME 04401

142

Asthma Resources Directory

Information In Print

Leonardo L. Leonidas, MD

"Nocturnal Asthma"
Available from:
National Jewish Center for
Immunology
and Respiratory Medicine
1400 Jackson at ColFax (APD)
Denver, CO 80206-2762
800-222-LUNG (5864)
In CO 303-355-LUNG (5864)
303-398-1907

"Occupational Asthma"
Available from:
Asthma & Allergy Foundation of
America
1125 15th St. N.W. #502 (APD)
Washington, DC 20005
202-466-7643
Fax 202-466-8940

"One Minute Asthma"
Thomas F. Plaut, MD
Pedipress, Inc.
125 Red Gate Ln. (APD)
Amherst, MA 01002
800-344-5864
413-549-7798

"Parent's Guide to Allergies & Asthma, A"
Marion Steinmann
Available from:
Delta Delacorte
Div. of Bantam Doubleday Dell
666th Ave. (APD)
New York, NY 10103
800-221-4676
212-765-6500

"Parent's Guide to Asthma, A: How You Can Help Your Child"
Nancy Sander
Available from:
Allergy & Asthma Network/
Mothers of Asthmatics, Inc.
3554 Chain Bridge Rd. Ste 200 (APD)
Fairfax, VA 22030-2709
Orders 800-878-4403

703-385-4403
Fax 703-352-4354
and:
Asthma Outreach Library
37 Pillsbury Rd. (APD)
Sandown, NH 03873
603-329-5301
and:
Doubleday & Co.
Div. of Bantam Doubleday Dell
666 Fifth Ave.
New York, NY 10103
800-223-6834 Ext. 479
NY 212-765-6500

"Patient's Guide to Asthma, A"
Fred Leffert, MD
Available from:
Allen & Hanburys™
Div. of Glaxo, Inc.
5 Moore Dr. (APD)
Research Triangle Park, NC 27709
919-248-2100
Medical services 919-248-2100

"Peak Flow Monitoring"
Available from:
Asthma & Allergy Foundation of
America
1125 15th St. N.W. #502 (APD)
Washington, DC 20005
202-466-7643
Fax 202-466-8940

"Peak Performance: A Strategy for Asthma Self-Assessment"
Guillermo R. Mendoza, MD
Available from:
Allergy & Asthma Network/
Mothers of Asthmatics, Inc.
3554 Chain Bridge Rd. Ste 200 (APD)
Fairfax, VA 22030-2709
Orders 800-878-4403
703-385-4403
Fax 703-352-4354
and:
Hawthorne Community Medical Group
2990 Sepulveda Blvd. (APD)
Los Angeles, CA 90064

Asthma Resources Directory

Information In Print

"Pollen Aeroallergens of the United States"
Available from:
Center Laboratories
35 Channel Dr. (APD)
PO Box 70 (APD)
Port Washington, NY 11050
Customer service 800-223-6837

"Pollen Allergy"
Available from:
National Institute of Allergy
& Infectious Diseases
NIH - Public Health Services
Bldg. 31 Rm. 72-32 (APD)
Public Health Services
9000 Rockville Pike
Bethesda, MD 20892-0001
301-496-5717
301-496-4000

"Practical Management of Asthma"
Arthur Dawson, Editor
Ronald A. Simon, Editor
Available from:
Grune & Stratton
Subs. of Harcourt Brace Jovanovich, Inc.
111 Fifth Ave. (APD)
New York, NY 10003
212-741-4888

"Questions and Answers about Asthma and Allergy"
Available from:
National Institute of Allergy
& Infectious Diseases
NIH - Public Health Services
Bldg. 31 Rm. 72-32 (APD)
Public Health Services
9000 Rockville Pike
Bethesda, MD 20892-0001
301-496-5717
301-496-4000

"Steroid Dependency in People with Asthma"
Available from:

Asthma & Allergy Foundation of America
1125 15th St. N.W. #502 (APD)
Washington, DC 20005
202-466-7643
Fax 202-466-8940

"Take Care of Yourself in an Emergency"
Available from:
American Allergy Assn.
1259 El Camino #254 (APD)
Menlo Park, CA 94025
415-322-1663
Internet AllergyAid@aol.com

"Taming Asthma and Allergy: Controlling Your Environent"
Robert A. Wood, MD
Available from:
Asthma & Allergy Foundation of America
1125 15th St. N.W. #502 (APD)
Washington, DC 20005
202-466-7643
Fax 202-466-8940

"There are Solutions for the Student with Asthma"
Available from:
American Lung Assn.
800-LUNG-USA (5864-872)
Refers to local ALA for information

"Understanding and Managing Asthma"
John L. Deker
Michael A. Kaliner
Available from:
Avon Books
Div. of Hearst Corp.(APD)
1350 Ave. of the Americas 2nd Flr.
New York, NY 10019
800-238-0658
212-261-6800

"Understanding Asthma: A Blueprint for Breathing"
Available from:

Asthma Resources Directory

Information In Print

Asthma & Allergy Foundation of America
1125 15th St. N.W. #502 (APD)
Washington, DC 20005
202-466-7643
Fax 202-466-8940

"Understanding the Immune System"
Available from:
National Institute of Allergy
& Infectious Diseases
NIH - Public Health Services
Bldg. 31 Rm. 72-32 (APD)
Public Health Services
9000 Rockville Pike
Bethesda, MD 20892-0001
301-496-5717
301-496-4000

Understanding Series
"Understanding Asthma,"
"Understanding Immunology"
Available from:
National Jewish Center for
Immunology
and Respiratory Medicine
1400 Jackson at ColFax (APD)
Denver, CO 80206-2762
800-222-LUNG (5864)
In CO 303-355-LUNG (5864)
303-398-1907

"Users' Guide to Peak Flow Monitoring"
Guillermo Mendoza, MD
Nancy Sander
Debra Scherrer
    English, Spanish
Available from:
Allergy & Asthma Network/
Mothers of Asthmatics, Inc.
3554 Chain Bridge Rd. Ste 200 (APD)
Fairfax, VA 22030-2709
Orders 800-878-4403
703-385-4403
Fax 703-352-4354
and:
Allergy Supply Co., Inc. The
11994 Star Court (APD)

Herndon, VA 22071
800-323-6744
Metropolitan DC 703-391-2011
Fax 703-391-2014
BBS 703-521-0638
and:
Asthma Outreach Library
37 Pillsbury Rd. (APD)
Sandown, NH 03873
603-329-5301

"Using Medicines Wisely"
Available from:
American Lung Assn.
800-LUNG-USA (5864-872)
Refers to local ALA for information

"What Americans Should Know About Asthma: Teacher's Guide"
Available from:
Allen & Hanburys™
Div. of Glaxo, Inc.
5 Moore Dr. (APD)
Research Triangle Park, NC 27709
919-248-2100
Medical services 919-248-2100

"What Every Educator Should Know About Asthma"
    Call American Lung Assn. of
Colorado for availability

"What Everyone Needs to Know About..."
    Separate Titles: Theophyline.
Corticosteroids (Spanish or English).
Cromolyn Sodium. Bronchodilators.
Asthma. Exercise-induced Asthma.
Rhinitis.
Available from:
Allergy & Asthma Network/
Mothers of Asthmatics, Inc.
3554 Chain Bridge Rd. Ste 200 (APD)
Fairfax, VA 22030-2709
Orders 800-878-4403
703-385-4403
Fax 703-352-4354

Asthma Resources Directory

Information In Print

"What Everyone Should Know About Asthma"
Available from:
American Lung Assn.
800-LUNG-USA (5864-872)
Refers to local ALA for information

"What You Can Do About Asthma"
Nathaniel Altman
Available from:
Dell Publishing Co., Inc.
Div. of Bantam Doubleday Dell Pub.
666 Fifth Ave. (APD)
New York, NY 10103

"What You Can Do About Asthma"
Nathaniel Altman
Available from:
Dell Publishing Co., Inc.
Div. of Bantam Doubleday Dell Pub.
666 Fifth Ave. (APD)
New York, NY 10103

"What You Need to Know About Asthma"
Michael A. Kaliner, MD
from Public Health Service NIH
Available from:
Boehringer Ingelheim Pharmaceuticals, Inc.
90 E. Ridge (APD)
PO Box 368 (APD)
Ridgefield, CT 06877
203-438-0311
and:
USDHHS - Public Health Service
National Institutes of Health
200 Independence Ave. SW Rm 716G (APD)
Washington, DC 20201-0001

"Women and Asthma"
Available from:
Asthma & Allergy Foundation of America
1125 15th St. N.W. #502 (APD)
Washington, DC 20005
202-466-7643

Fax 202-466-8940

"You Can Control Asthma"
Available from:
Center for Interdisciplinary
Research on Immunologic Diseases
Georgetown Univ. School of Medicine
3900 Reservoir Rd. N.W. (APD)
Washington, DC 20007

"Your Asthma Answer Book"
Available from:
Demos Publications
156 Fifth Ave. Ste 1018 (APD)
New York, NY 10010
212-255-8768

"Your Child and Asthma"
Available from:
National Jewish Center for Immunology
and Respiratory Medicine
1400 Jackson at ColFax (APD)
Denver, CO 80206-2762
800-222-LUNG (5864)
In CO 303-355-LUNG (5864)
303-398-1907

"Your Child and Asthma"
Available from:
National Jewish Center for Immunology
and Respiratory Medicine
1400 Jackson at ColFax (APD)
Denver, CO 80206-2762
800-222-LUNG (5864)
In CO 303-355-LUNG (5864)
303-398-1907

"Your Child's Lungs are for Life"
Available from:
American Lung Assn.
800-LUNG-USA (5864-872)
Refers to local ALA for information

"Your Indoor Environment"
Available from:
American Allergy Assn.
1259 El Camino #254 (APD)
Menlo Park, CA 94025

146

Asthma Resources Directory

Information In Print

415-322-1663
Internet AllergyAid@aol.com

"Your Working Lungs Part 1: Description, Function, Problem Pollutants"
FDA
Available from:
American Allergy Assn.
1259 El Camino #254 (APD)
Menlo Park, CA 94025
415-322-1663
Internet AllergyAid@aol.com

"Your Working Lungs Part 2: Diseases, Examination, Treatment"
FDA
Available from:
American Allergy Assn.
1259 El Camino #254 (APD)
Menlo Park, CA 94025
415-322-1663
Internet AllergyAid@aol.com

OF RELATED INTEREST

"Take Care with Over-the-Counter Asthma Medicine"
Available from:
Nonprescription Drug Manufacturers Assn.
NDMA
1150 Connecticut Ave. NW (APD)
Washington, DC 20036
202-429-9260
Fax 202-223-6835

IN PRINT IN SPANISH

"Asma en un Minuto, El"
Thomas F. Plaut, MD
Available from:
Pedipress, Inc.
125 Red Gate Lane (APD)
Amherst, MA 01002

"Como Controlar El Asma"
(Spanish language version of "Controlling Asthma")
Available from:
American Lung Assn.
800-LUNG-USA (5864-872)
Refers to local ALA for information

"Get a Check-up for Your Car!"
(in Spanish)
Available from:
American Lung Assn.
800-LUNG-USA (5864-872)
Refers to local ALA for information

"Home Indoor Air Quality Checklist" (in Spanish)
Available from:
American Lung Assn.
800-LUNG-USA (5864-872)
Refers to local ALA for information

"Lo Que Usted Debe Saber Acerca Del Asma"
Available from:
USDHHS - Public Health Service
National Institutes of Health
200 Independence Ave. SW Rm 716G (APD)
Washington, DC 20201-0001

"Manual Sobre Asma"
("The Asthma Handbook" in Spanish)
Available from:
American Lung Assn.
800-LUNG-USA (5864-872)
Refers to local ALA for information

"Peak Flow Meter Monitoring in Spanish"
Available from:
HealthScan Products, Inc.
908 Pompton Ave. (APD)
Cedar Grove, NJ 07009-1292
800-962-1266
In NJ 201-857-3414

"Users' Guide to Peak Flow Monitoring"
Guillermo Mendoza, MD

147

Asthma Resources Directory

Information In Print

Nancy Sander
Debra Scherrer
    Spanish
Available from:
Allergy & Asthma Network/
Mothers of Asthmatics, Inc.
3554 Chain Bridge Rd. Ste 200 (APD)
Fairfax, VA 22030-2709
Orders 800-878-4403
703-385-4403
Fax 703-352-4354
and:
Asthma Outreach Library
37 Pillsbury Rd. (APD)
Sandown, NH 03873
603-329-5301

"What Everyone Needs to Know About Corticosteroids"
In Spanish
Available from:
Allergy & Asthma Network/
Mothers of Asthmatics, Inc.
3554 Chain Bridge Rd. Ste 200 (APD)
Fairfax, VA 22030-2709
Orders 800-878-4403
703-385-4403
Fax 703-352-4354

"What Everyone Needs to Know About Theophyline"
In Spanish
Available from:
Allergy & Asthma Network/
Mothers of Asthmatics, Inc.
3554 Chain Bridge Rd. Ste 200 (APD)
Fairfax, VA 22030-2709
Orders 800-878-4403
703-385-4403
Fax 703-352-4354

IN PRINT FOR CHILDREN

"ABC of Asthma"
John Rees, Bristish Medical
Association
Available from:
Taylor & Francis, Inc.
79 Madison Ave. (APD)

New York, NY 10016
800-821-8312
212-725-1999

"All About Asthma"
William Ostrow
Vivian Ostrow
Available from:
Albert Whitman & Co.
5747 W. Howard St. (APD)
Niles, IL 60648
708-647-1355

"Asthma and You"
Chris Mulligan, RN, MS, ANP
Victoria S. Simpson, RN, PNP
Available from:
Allen & Hanburys™
Div. of Glaxo, Inc.
5 Moore Dr. (APD)
Research Triangle Park, NC 27709
919-248-2100
Medical services 919-248-2100

"Asthma Attack by Bo B. Bear, The"
Charlotte L. Casterline, MD
Available from:
Asthma Outreach Library
37 Pillsbury Rd. (APD)
Sandown, NH 03873
603-329-5301
and:
Info-All Book Co.
5 Old Well Ln. (APD)
Dallas, PA 18612

"Becky's Story"
(For siblings of hospitalized children)
D. Baznik
Available from:
Assn. for Care of Children's Health
7910 Woodmont Ave. #300 (APD)
Bethesda, MD 20814-3015
301-654-6549
Fax 301-986-4553

"Best of SuperStuff for Kids with Asthma"
Available from:

Asthma Resources Directory

Information In Print

American Lung Assn.
800-LUNG-USA (5864-872)
Refers to local ALA for information

"Captain America Meets the Asthma Monster"
Comic book
Available from:
Allen & Hanburys™
Div. of Glaxo, Inc.
5 Moore Dr. (APD)
Research Triangle Park, NC 27709
919-248-2100
Medical services 919-248-2100
and:
Asthma Outreach Library
37 Pillsbury Rd. (APD)
Sandown, NH 03873
603-329-5301

"Captain America: Return of the Asthma Monster"
Comic book
Available from:
Allen & Hanburys™
Div. of Glaxo, Inc.
5 Moore Dr. (APD)
Research Triangle Park, NC 27709
919-248-2100
Medical services 919-248-2100
and:
Asthma Outreach Library
37 Pillsbury Rd. (APD)
Sandown, NH 03873
603-329-5301

"Captain Wonderlung: Breathing Exercises for Asthmatic Children"
Comic book style
Available from:
American Academy of Pediatrics
141 Northwest Point Blvd (APD)
Elk Grove Village, IL 60007-1098
PO Box 927 (APD)
Elk Grove Village, IL 60009-0927
708-228-5005
Fax 708-228-5097
and:
Asthma Outreach Library
37 Pillsbury Rd. (APD)

Sandown, NH 03873
603-329-5301

"Child Goes to the Hospital, A"
Available from:
Assn. for Care of Children's Health
7910 Woodmont Ave. #300 (APD)
Bethesda, MD 20814-3015
301-654-6549
Fax 301-986-4553

"David, Anne and the Asthma Monster"
Sandoz
    Ask your doctor about availability

Forest Friends
Coloring book on asthma triggers
Available from:
American Assn. for Respiratory Care
11030 Ables Ln. (APD)
Dallas, TX 75229-4593
214-243-2272
Fax 214-484-2720

"Going to the Hospital"
Available from:
Assn. for Care of Children's Health
7910 Woodmont Ave. #300 (APD)
Bethesda, MD 20814-3015
301-654-6549
Fax 301-986-4553

"I'm A Meter Reader"
Nancy Sander
    English or Spanish
Available from:
Allen & Hanburys™
Div. of Glaxo, Inc.
5 Moore Dr. (APD)
Research Triangle Park, NC 27709
919-248-2100
Medical services 919-248-2100
and:
Allergy & Asthma Network/
Mothers of Asthmatics, Inc.
3554 Chain Bridge Rd. Ste 200 (APD)
Fairfax, VA 22030-2709
Orders 800-878-4403
703-385-4403

149

Asthma Resources Directory

Information In Print

Fax 703-352-4354
and:
Asthma Outreach Library
37 Pillsbury Rd. (APD)
Sandown, NH 03873
603-329-5301

"Lion Who Had Asthma, The"

Jonathan London
Available from:
Albert Whitman & Co.
5747 W. Howard St. (APD)
Niles, IL 60648
708-647-1355
and:
Asthma & Allergy Foundation of
America
1125 15th St. N.W. #502 (APD)
Washington, DC 20005
202-466-7643
Fax 202-466-8940

"Luke Has Asthma, Too"

Alison Rogers
Available from:
Allergy Asthma Technology
4151 N. Kedzie (APD)
PO Box 18398 (APD)
Chicago, IL 60618
800-621-5545
312-465-8020
Fax 312-465-7619
and:
Waterfront Books
98 Brookes Ave. (APD)
Burlington, VT 05401
802-638-7477
800-456-7500 Ext. 2000

"My Friend Has Asthma"

Charlotte Casterline, MD
Available from:
Asthma Outreach Library
37 Pillsbury Rd. (APD)
Sandown, NH 03873
603-329-5301
and:
Info-All Book Co.
5 Old Well Ln. (APD)
Dallas, PA 18612

"No Smoking Coloring Book"

Available from:
American Lung Assn.
800-LUNG-USA (5864-872)
Refers to local ALA for information

"Sam the Allergen"

Charlotte Casterline, MD
Available from:
Asthma Outreach Library
37 Pillsbury Rd. (APD)
Sandown, NH 03873
603-329-5301
and:
Info-All Book Co.
5 Old Well Ln. (APD)
Dallas, PA 18612

"Sneezing Wheezing Santa, The"

Melvyn Wolk, MD
Coloring book
Available from
Melvin Wolk, MD
PO Box 772 (APD)
Waverly, PA 18471
Available from:
Asthma Outreach Library
37 Pillsbury Rd. (APD)
Sandown, NH 03873
603-329-5301

"So You Have Asthma, Too!"

Nancy Sander
    English or Spanish
Available from:
Allen & Hanburys™
Div. of Glaxo, Inc.
5 Moore Dr. (APD)
Research Triangle Park, NC 27709
919-248-2100
Medical services 919-248-2100
and:
Allergy & Asthma Network/
Mothers of Asthmatics, Inc.
3554 Chain Bridge Rd. Ste 200 (APD)
Fairfax, VA 22030-2709
Orders 800-878-4403
703-385-4403
Fax 703-352-4354
and:

Asthma Resources Directory

Information In Print

Asthma Outreach Library
37 Pillsbury Rd. (APD)
Sandown, NH 03873
603-329-5301

"Spiderman Battles the Myth Monster!"
Marvel comic book
Available from:
Asthma & Allergy Foundation of
America
1125 15th St. N.W. #502 (APD)
Washington, DC 20005
202-466-7643
Fax 202-466-8940

"Teaching Myself About Asthma"
G. Parcel
K. Tiernan
P. Nader, et. al.
Available from:
Asthma & Allergy Foundation of
America
1125 15th St. N.W. #502 (APD)
Washington, DC 20005
202-466-7643
Fax 202-466-8940
and:
Asthma Outreach Library
37 Pillsbury Rd. (APD)
Sandown, NH 03873
603-329-5301
and:
Health Education Associates
14 North Lake Rd. (APD)
Columbia, SC 29223

"Thin Air"
David Getz
Available from:
Henry Holt & Co.
115 W. 18th St. (APD)
New York, NY 10011
NY 212-886-9200
800-247-3912

"Winning over Asthma"
Eileen Dolan Savage
Coloring book
Available from:

Allergy Asthma Technology
4151 N. Kedzie (APD)
PO Box 18398 (APD)
Chicago, IL 60618
800-621-5545
312-465-8020
Fax 312-465-7619
and:
Asthma & Allergy Foundation of
America
1125 15th St. N.W. #502 (APD)
Washington, DC 20005
202-466-7643
Fax 202-466-8940
and:
Asthma Outreach Library
37 Pillsbury Rd. (APD)
Sandown, NH 03873
603-329-5301
and:
Charles B. Stack, Inc.
6900 Grove Rd. (APD)
Thorofare, NJ 08036
800-257-8290
NJ 609-848-1000
and:
Dolan Press
1645 Gales Ct. (APD)
Forest Grove, OR 97116
503-357-7682

IN SPANISH FOR CHILDREN

"I'm A Meter Reader"
Nancy Sander
    English or Spanish
Available from:
Allen & Hanburys™
Div. of Glaxo, Inc.
5 Moore Dr. (APD)
Research Triangle Park, NC 27709
919-248-2100
Medical services 919-248-2100
and:
Allergy & Asthma Network/
Mothers of Asthmatics, Inc.
3554 Chain Bridge Rd. Ste 200 (APD)
Fairfax, VA 22030-2709
Orders 800-878-4403

Asthma Resources Directory

Information In Print

703-385-4403
Fax 703-352-4354
and:
Asthma Outreach Library
37 Pillsbury Rd. (APD)
Sandown, NH 03873
603-329-5301

OF RELATED INTEREST FOR CHILDREN

"Emergency Room: An ABC Tour"
Available from:
Pediatric Projects, Inc.
PO Box 1880 (APD)
Santa Monica, CA 90406

"Hospital Game, The"
E. Crocker
Available from:
Assn. for Care of Children's Health
7910 Woodmont Ave. #300 (APD)
Bethesda, MD 20814-3015
301-654-6549
Fax 301-986-4553

"Hospital Story: A Book for Children and Parents Together"
Available from:
Pediatric Projects, Inc.
PO Box 1880 (APD)
Santa Monica, CA 90406

"I'll Never Love Anything Again"
Judy Dalton
Available from:
Albert Whitman & Co.
5747 W. Howard St. (APD)
Niles, IL 60648
708-647-1355

"Let's Talk About Going to the Hospital"
Available from:
Health Edco, Inc.
PO Box 21207 (APD)
Waco, TX 76702-1207
817-776-6461

800-433-2677

IN PRINT FOR TEENS

AAFA Teen Support Groups
written by teens across the country
Available from:
Asthma & Allergy Foundation of America
1125 15th St. N.W. #502 (APD)
Washington, DC 20005
202-466-7643
Fax 202-466-8940

"Let's Talk About Asthma: A Guide for Teens"
Available from:
American Lung Assn.
800-LUNG-USA (5864-872)
Refers to local ALA for information

"Reaching for the Stars. Teens Talk to Teens About Asthma"
Available from:
Asthma & Allergy Foundation of America
1125 15th St. N.W. #502 (APD)
Washington, DC 20005
202-466-7643
Fax 202-466-8940

"Teens and Asthma"
Available from:
American Lung Assn.
800-LUNG-USA (5864-872)
Refers to local ALA for information
and:
Asthma & Allergy Foundation of America
1125 15th St. N.W. #502 (APD)
Washington, DC 20005
202-466-7643
Fax 202-466-8940

"Teens Face to Face with Chronic Illness"
Suzanne LeVert
Available from:

152

Asthma Resources Directory

Information In Print

Asthma & Allergy Foundation of America
1125 15th St. N.W. #502 (APD)
Washington, DC 20005
202-466-7643
Fax 202-466-8940

OF RELATED INTEREST FOR TEENS

"For Teenagers: Your Stay in the Hospital"
Available from:
Assn. for Care of Children's Health
7910 Woodmont Ave. #300 (APD)
Bethesda, MD 20814-3015
301-654-6549
Fax 301-986-4553

"Hospital Journal"
Available from:
Assn. for Care of Children's Health
7910 Woodmont Ave. #300 (APD)
Bethesda, MD 20814-3015
301-654-6549
Fax 301-986-4553

IN PRINT FOR PROFESSIONALS

American Lung Assn. Reprints
Call your local ALA branch for reprints of the following articles:
"Randomized Trial of A.C.T. (Asthma Care Training) for Kids, A"
C.E. Lewis, MD et. al.
"School Health Education Program for Children with Asthma Aged 8-11 Years, A"
D. Evans, et. al.
"Asthma Education: A National Strategy" (NHLBI & NIAID)
S.R. Parker, et. al.
"Asthma Self-Management Education Research and Implications for Clinical Practice
N.M. Clark, et. al.

"Asthma Self-Management Programs: Premises not Promises
E.L. Klingelhofer, et. al.
"Collaborative Asthma Self-Management Evaluation Designs"
M.C. Hindi-Alexander, et. al.
"Living with Asthma: Replications and Extensions"
T.L. Creer
"Making Childhood Asthma Management Education Happen in the Community: Translating Health Behavioral Research into Local Programs"
C.B. Krutzsch
"Managing Better: Children, Parents, and Asthma"
N.M. Clark, et. al.
"Self-Management Education of Children with Asthma: Air Wise"
W.L. McNabb, et. al.
"The Impact of Health Education on Frequency and Cost of Health Care Used by Low Income Children with Asthma"
N.M. Clark, et. al.
"The Role of Patient Education in the Management of Childhood Asthma"
S.R. Wilson-Pessano
"Workshop on Asthma Self-Management, Summary of Workshop Discussion"
S.R. Wilson-Pessano, et. al.
Available from:
American Lung Assn.
800-LUNG-USA (5864-872)
Refers to local ALA for information

ATS reprints on office practice
"Essentials of a Pulmonary Consultation"
"Quality Assurance in Pulmony Function Laboratories"
"Standardization of Spirometry"
Available from:
American Lung Assn.
800-LUNG-USA (5864-872)
Refers to local ALA for information

Asthma Resources Directory

Information In Print

"Allergic Diseases"
Roy Patterson, MD
Lippincott Medical
Available from:
Harper & Row, Publishers, Inc.
10 E. 53rd St.
New York, NY 10022
212-207-7000
800-242-7737

"Allergy Products Directory"
Controlling Your Environment
Allergy/Asthma Finding Help
Asthma Resources Directory
Food Allergy Resources
Available from:
Allergy Publications
1259 El Camino #254 (APD)
Menlo Park, CA 94025
415-322-1663

"Allergy: Principles and Practice"
E. Middleton, Jr., Editor
Available from:
C.V. Mosby Co.
Subs. of Times Mirror Co.
11830 Westline Industrial Dr. (APD)
PO Box 46908 (APD)
St. Louis, MO 63146-9988
800-325-4177
MO 314-872-8370
Orders 800-426-4545

"Allergy: Theory and Practice"
Phillip E. Korenblat, MD, Editor
H. James Wedner, MD, Editor
Available from:
Grune & Stratton
Subs. of Harcourt Brace Jovanovich, Inc.
111 Fifth Ave. (APD)
New York, NY 10003
212-741-4888

"Asthma & Allergy in Pregnancy & Early Infancy"
Michael Schatz, MD, Editor
Robert S. Zeiger, MD, Editor
Available from:

Marcel Dekker, Inc.
270 Madison Ave. (APD)
800-228-1160
NY 212-696-9000

"Asthma as an Inflammatory Disease"
O'Byrne, Editor
Available from:
Sterling Publishing Co., Inc.
387 Park Ave. S. (APD)
New York, NY 10016-8810
NY 212-532-7160
800-367-9692

"Asthma Care and Patient Information: The Nurse's Role"
Christine W. Wagner, RN
Available from:
Asthma & Allergy Foundation of America
1125 15th St. N.W. #502 (APD)
Washington, DC 20005
202-466-7643
Fax 202-466-8940

"Asthma Drugs Theory and Practice"
Jenne & Murphy
Available from:
Marcel Dekker, Inc.
270 Madison Ave. (APD)
800-228-1160
NY 212-696-9000

"Asthma in the Workplace"
Bernstein, et al.
Available from:
Marcel Dekker, Inc.
270 Madison Ave. (APD)
800-228-1160
NY 212-696-9000

"Asthma Pathophysiology and Treatment"
Tinkelman, et. al.
Available from:
Marcel Dekker, Inc.
270 Madison Ave. (APD)
800-228-1160

Asthma Resources Directory

Information In Print

NY 212-696-9000

"Asthma Therapy: A Behavioral Health Care System for Respiratory Disorders"
Thomas L. Creer
Available from:
Springer Publishing Co.
536 Broadway (APD)
New York, NY 10012
212-431-4370

"Asthma"
T.J. Clark, MD
Available from:
Van Nostrand Reinhold
Div. of The Thomson Corp.
115 Fifth Ave. (APD)
New York, NY 10003
800-242-7737
212-254-3232

"Asthma: A Practical Guide for Physicians"
Available from:
American Lung Assn.
800-LUNG-USA (5864-872)
Refers to local ALA for information

"Asthma: Basic Mechanisms & Clinical Management"
P.J. Barnes, MD et al., Editors
Available from:
Academic Press, Inc.
Subs. of Harcourt Brace Jovanovich, Inc.
465 S. Lincoln Dr. (APD)
Troy, MI 63379
619-231-6616
800-346-8648

"Asthma Physiology, Immunopharmacology & Treatment"
Barry A. Kray, et. al., Editors
Available from:
Academic Press, Inc.
Subs. of Harcourt Brace Jovanovich, Inc.
465 S. Lincoln Dr. (APD)

Troy, MI 63379
619-231-6616
800-346-8648

"Bronchial Asthma"
E.B. Weiss, Editor
M.S. Segal, Editor
M. Stein, Editor
Available from:
Little, Brown & Co.
Div. of Time, Inc.
34 Beacon St. (APD)
Boston, MA 02108
800-343-9204
MA 617-227-0730

"Bronchial Asthma: Mechanisms & Therapeutics"
Earle B. Weiss, MD, Editor
Myron Stein, MD, Editor
Available from:
Little, Brown & Co.
Div. of Time, Inc.
34 Beacon St. (APD)
Boston, MA 02108
800-343-9204
MA 617-227-0730

"Childhood Asthma: Pathophysiology & Treatment"
David G. Tinkelman, MD, Editor
Charles K. Naspitz, MD, Editor
Available from:
Marcel Dekker, Inc.
270 Madison Ave. (APD)
800-228-1160
NY 212-696-9000

"Clinical Strategies in Adult Asthma"
Charles H. Scoggin
Thomas L. Petty
Available from:
Lea & Febiger
200 Chester Field Pkwy. (APD)
Malvern, PA 19355-9725
800-444-1785
215-251-2230

Asthma Resources Directory

Information In Print

"Consumer Guide for Room Air Cleaners"
Available from:
Assn. of Home Appliance Manufacturers
AHAM
20 N. Wacker Dr. (APD)
Chicago, IL 60606
312-984-5800

"Current Perspectives in the Immunology of Respiratory Diseases"
A.B. Kay, Editor
Edward J. Goetzl, Editor
Available from:
Churchill Livingstone, Inc.
650 Ave. of the Americas (APD)
New York, NY 10011
800-553-5462
212-206-5000
Fax 212-727-7808
Customer Service 800-503-5426
and
Churchill Livingstone, Inc.
128 Long Acre (APD)
London, WC25 9AN
United Kingdom
011-44-71836-5852

"Current Therapy in Allergy, Immunology, and Rheumatology"
Lawrence M. Lichtenstein, MD, PhD
Anthony S. Fauci, MD
Available from:
C.V. Mosby Co.
Subs. of Times Mirror Co.
11830 Westline Industrial Dr. (APD)
PO Box 46908 (APD)
St. Louis, MO 63146-9988
800-325-4177
MO 314-872-8370
Orders 800-426-4545

"Current Treatment of Ambulatory Asthma"
Guy A. Settipane, MD, Editor
Available from:
New England & Regional Allergy Proceedings

95 Pitman St. (APD)
Providence, RI 02906

"Drugs for the Respiratory System"
Reuben M. Cherniack, MD
Available from:
Grune & Stratton
Subs. of Harcourt Brace Jovanovich, Inc.
111 Fifth Ave. (APD)
New York, NY 10003
212-741-4888

"Eosinophils in Asthma & Allergy"
A.B. Kay, MD
Available from:
Blackwell Scientific Pubns., Inc.
238 Main St. (APD)
Cambridge, MA 02142
800-445-6638
617-225-0430

"Eosinophils in Asthma"
J. Morley, Editor
I. Colditz, Editor
Available from:
Academic Press, Inc.
Subs. of Harcourt Brace Jovanovich, Inc.
465 S. Lincoln Dr. (APD)
Troy, MI 63379
619-231-6616
800-346-8648

"Evaluation and Management of Allergic and Asthmatic Disorders"
Eric Gershwin
Stephen M. Nagy, Editor
Available from:
Grune & Stratton
Subs. of Harcourt Brace Jovanovich, Inc.
111 Fifth Ave. (APD)
New York, NY 10003
212-741-4888

156

Asthma Resources Directory

Information In Print

"Guide to Atmospheric Pollen Counting and Differentiation"
Available from:
Center Laboratories
35 Channel Dr. (APD)
PO Box 70 (APD)
Port Washington, NY 11050
Customer service 800-223-6837

"Guide to Bronchial Asthma, A"
H.A. Herxheimer
Available from:
Academic Press, Inc.
Subs. of Harcourt Brace Jovanovich, Inc.
465 S. Lincoln Dr. (APD)
Troy, MI 63379
619-231-6616
800-346-8648

"Guidelines for the Diagnosis and Management of Asthma"
Available from:
Asthma Information Center
Nat'l Heart, Lung & Blood Inst.
4733 Bethesda Ave. #530 (APD)
Bethedsda, MD 20814
301-951-3260
and:
National Institutes of Health
9000 Rockville Pike (APD)
Bethesda, MD 20892-0001
301-496-4000
Fax 301-496-2443

"Lung Function Assessment & Applications in Medicine"
J.E. Cotes, MD
G.L. Leathart, MD
Available from:
Blackwell Scientific Pubns., Inc.
238 Main St. (APD)
Cambridge, MA 02142
800-445-6638
617-225-0430

"Manual of Allergy and Immunology, The"
Glenn Lawlor, MD, Editor
Thomas Fischer, MD, Editor
Available from:
Little, Brown & Co.
Div. of Time, Inc.
34 Beacon St. (APD)
Boston, MA 02108
800-343-9204
MA 617-227-0730

"Manual of Clinical Problems in Asthma, Allergy & Related Disorders, A"
Don A. Bukstein
Robert C. Strunk
Available from:
Little, Brown & Co.
Div. of Time, Inc.
34 Beacon St. (APD)
Boston, MA 02108
800-343-9204
MA 617-227-0730

"Manual of Pulmonary Function Testing"
Ruppel
Available from:
C.V. Mosby Co.
Subs. of Times Mirror Co.
11830 Westline Industrial Dr. (APD)
PO Box 46908 (APD)
St. Louis, MO 63146-9988
800-325-4177
MO 314-872-8370
Orders 800-426-4545

"New Developments in the Therapy of Allergic Disorders & Asthma"
S.A. Langer, MD
Available from:
S. Karger, AG
26 W. Avon Rd. (APD)
Box 529 (APD)
Farmington, CT 06085
203-675-7834

"Nocturnal Asthma"
P.J. Barnes
J. Levy, Editor
Available from:
Longwood Publishing Group, Inc.

157

Asthma Resources Directory

Information In Print

Stoneham Rd. (APD)
PO Box 757 (APD)
Wakefield, NH 03872
603-522-6303

"Occupational Asthma"
Emil J. Bardana, Jr., MD et al.
Available from:
Hanley & Belfus, Inc.
Dist. by C.V. Mosby Co.
210 S. 13th St. (APD)
Philadelphia, PA 19107
215-546-7293

Professional Materials
"Anticipatory Counseling" (asthma counseling in community health centers)
"Personal Protection Against Air Pollution - The Physicians Role"
Available from:
American Lung Assn.
800-LUNG-USA (5864-872)
Refers to local ALA for information

"Pulmonary Function Testing: A Practical Approach"
Jack Wanger, MD
Available from:
Williams & Wilkins Co.
428 E. Preston St. (APD)
Baltimore, MD 21202
800-638-0672
MD 301-528-4000

"Pulmonary Function Testing: Guidelines and Controversies"
Jack L. Clausen, MD, Editor
L. Powell Zarins, Editor
Available from:
Grune & Stratton
Subs. of Harcourt Brace Jovanovich, Inc.
111 Fifth Ave. (APD)
New York, NY 10003
212-741-4888

"Pulmonary Function Testing: Indications and Interpretations"
Archie F. Wilson, MD, PhD, Editor
Available from:

Grune & Stratton
Subs. of Harcourt Brace Jovanovich, Inc.
111 Fifth Ave. (APD)
New York, NY 10003
212-741-4888

"Pulmonary Function Testing: Principles & Practice"
Stephen A. Conrad et al., Editors
Available from:
Churchill Livingstone, Inc.
650 Ave. of the Americas (APD)
New York, NY 10011
800-553-5462
212-206-5000
Fax 212-727-7808
Customer Service 800-503-5426
and
Churchill Livingstone, Inc.
128 Long Acre (APD)
London, WC25 9AN
United Kingdom
011-44-71836-5852

"Pulmonary Function Tests in Clinical and Occupational Lung Disease"
Albert A. Miller, MD, Editor
Available from:
Grune & Stratton
Subs. of Harcourt Brace Jovanovich, Inc.
111 Fifth Ave. (APD)
New York, NY 10003
212-741-4888

"Respiratory Distress Syndrome"
Kari O. Raivio
Nilo Hallman
Kauko Kouvalainen
Ilka Valimaki
Available from:
Academic Press, Inc.
Subs. of Harcourt Brace Jovanovich, Inc.
465 S. Lincoln Dr. (APD)
Troy, MI 63379
619-231-6616
800-346-8648

Asthma Resources Directory

Information In Print

"Respiratory Therapy Equipment"
McPherson & Spearman
Available from:
C.V. Mosby Co.
Subs. of Times Mirror Co.
11830 Westline Industrial Dr. (APD)
PO Box 46908 (APD)
St. Louis, MO 63146-9988
800-325-4177
MO 314-872-8370
Orders 800-426-4545

"Rhinitis and Asthma: Similarities and Differences"
Niels Mygind, MD
Ronald Dahl, MD
Ulf Pipkorn, MD
Available from:
C.V. Mosby Co.
Subs. of Times Mirror Co.
11830 Westline Industrial Dr. (APD)
PO Box 46908 (APD)
St. Louis, MO 63146-9988
800-325-4177
MO 314-872-8370
Orders 800-426-4545

"Standards for the Diagnosis and Care of Patients with Chronic Obstructive Pulmonary Disease (COPD) and Asthma"
American Lung Assn.
800-LUNG-USA (5864-872)
Refers to local ALA for information

"Sustained Release Theophylline and Nocturnal Asthma" vol 18
A.F. Isles, Editor
P. von Wichert, Editor
Available from:

Available from:
S. Karger, AG
26 W. Avon Rd. (APD)
Box 529 (APD)
Farmington, CT 06085
203-675-7834

"Theoretical and Clinical Aspects of Allergic Diseases"
H. Bostrom, Editor
N. Ljungstedt. Editor
Available from:
Coronet Books
311 Bainbridge St. (APD)
Philadelphia, PA 19147
215-925-5083

"Update on Childhood Asthma"
M.H. Schoni, MD, Editor
R. Kraemer, MD, Editor
Available from:
St. Martin's Press, Inc.
175 Fifth Ave. (APD)
New York, NY 10010

OF RELATED INTEREST
"Take Care with Over-the-Counter Asthma Medicine"
Available from:
Nonprescription Drug Manufacturers Assn.
NDMA
1150 Connecticut Ave. NW (APD)
Washington, DC 20036
202-429-9260
Fax 202-223-6835

Allergy Products Directory
Copyrighted. Reproduction Prohibited by Law. 1259 El Camino #254,Menlo Park, CA 94025

Asthma Resources Directory
Clearinghouses, Support Groups

CLEARINGHOUSES AND SUPPORT GROUPS

Not therapy groups and not a substitute for your doctor, self-help groups are composed of individuals with a common concern, illness, or experience that bring them together to receive and to give support to one another in dealing with day-to-day problems. Their main goal is to help their members to help themselves.

THE ROLE OF CLEARINGHOUSES

Clearinghouses will either put you in touch with a group in your area that deals with asthma or will try to match you with other families and help you form a local, mutual support group.

If clearinghouse aid is unavailable, try the telephone book, your local hospital, or social service agency; sometimes meetings are listed in the community bulletin board secions of your local newspapers or at the local community activities center.

Some clearinghouses provide directories or lists of existing grouops and can also provide information about local groups and pamphlets that tell you what to look for in a group and suggestions on how to start new groups.

WHAT TO EXPECT FROM A SUPPORT GROUP

As a member of a self-help or support group, you gain from being with others who share your problem. You can expect to learn more about allergies and asthma, exchange information about dealing with problems, and, perhaps, most importantly, learn that you are not alone with your fears, your anger, and your frustration.

Information gives you power. It allows for greater control in your life; problems don't seem so overwhelming. With your new knowledge and abilities, you may find that you feel better, cope better, and develop an increasing sense of satisfaction in your handling of difficult situations.

Be sure that there is a professional or knowledgeable and experienced advisor so that information you receive is correct. Avoid groups that seem centered on one solution or advise you to change your doctor's treatment. Support

160

Allergy Products Directory
Copyrighted. Reproduction Prohibited by Law. 1259 El Camino #254, Menlo Park, CA 94025

Asthma Resources Directory
Clearinghouses, Support Groups

groups should have a minimal cost, mainly for refreshments and should **not** be selling "cures."

Today's society is a fluid one and you may find that self-help groups reflect that fluidity.

If the one you call is no longer active, don't be discouraged. Try calling previous participants and bringing together other families you may know or have met at your own doctor's office.

Ask your doctor if he or she knows of an ongoing group or of some families who may be interested in starting one. Sometimes a notice posted in the waiting room of your doctor's office can be the start of a committed group.

FIRST STEP IN STARTING A SUPPORT GROUP

"Support Group Manual"
Nancy Sander
Allergy and Asthma Network
800-878-4403

"How to Organize a Self-Help Group"
National Self-Help Clearinghouse
212-642-2944

"Starting and Operating Support Groups"
National Resource Center for Family Support Programs
Family Resource Coalition
200 S. Michigan Ave. #1520
Chicago, IL 60604

"Support Group Resources Kit"
Nancy Sanker, OTR
Asthma and Allergy Foundation of America
202-466-7643

HELP US TO HELP YOU

When writing to the companies and organizations listed here, be sure to use the initials (APD) as part of the address and tell them you saw them listed in *Allergy Products Directory*.

If you call, be sure to tell them you found them in *Allergy Products Directory*.

Asthma Resources Directory

Clearinghouses

CLEARINGHOUSES

NATIONAL CLEARINGHOUSES

American Self-Help Clearinghouse
Information on self-help groups;
directory of self-help organizations
St. Clares-Riverside Med. Center
25 Pocono Rd. (APD)
Denville, NJ 07834
201-625-7101

California Self-Help Center
Information on health topics;
makes referrals to local, regional,
national organizations directly or
through reference books
California Self-Help Center
(Regional)
University of CA, Los Angeles
405 Hilgard Ave. (APD)
2349 Franz Hall
Los Angeles, CA 90024
In CA 800-222-LINK (5465)

Center for Self Help
Information on self-help resources
in caller's area
Center for Self-Help
Riverwood Center
PO Box 547 (APD)
Benton Harbor, MI 49022-0547
800-336-0341 local

Consumer Health Information Resource Institute
Referrals to local, regional, and
national organizations; faxes answers
to questions; does bibliographical
searches for a fee; book and resource
catalogue by mail; 9:00 am to 5:00 pm
central; M-F; patient education library;
sources of health information on
medical conditions, medications
Consumer Health Information
Research Institute
3521 Broadway (APD)
Kansas City, MO 64111

800-821-6671
MO 816-753-8850
Fax 816-753-6706

National Information Clearinghouse
for Infants with Disabilities
(Birth through three)
National Information System
Clearinghouse
CDD/USC
Benson Bldg. First Floor
1244 Blossom St. (APD)
Columbia, SC 29208
800-922-9234 Ext. 201 Voice & TDD
In SC 800-922-1107 Voice & TDD
Administrative 803-777-4435

National Maternal & Child Health Clearinghouse
Publications and referrals
8201 Greensboro Dr. #600 (APD)
McLean, VA 22102
703-821-8955 Ext. 254, 265

National Self-Help Clearinghouse
25 W. 43rd St. Rm. 620 (APD)
New York, NY 10036
212-642-2944
NY City Referrals 212-586-5770
Fax 212-719-2488

REGIONAL CLEARINGHOUSES

CALIFORNIA

Bay Area Self-Help Clearinghouse
Eleven counties in northern
California
Mental Health Assn. of San Francisco
2398 Pine St. (APD)
San Francisco, CA 94115
415-921-4044

Asthma Resources Directory

Clearinghouses

California Self-Help Center
Univ. of California, Los Angeles
405 Hilgard Ave. (APD)
2349 Franz Hall
Los Angeles, CA 90024
In CA: 800-222-LINK (5465)
213-825-1799

Tri-County Clearinghouse
Placer, Yolo, Sacramento
211 E. St. Ste. 5 (APD)
PO Box 447 (APD)
Davis, CA 95617
916-756-8181

CONNECTICUT
Connecticut Self-Help/Mutual Support Network
Consultation Ctr.
389 Whitney Ave. (APD)
New Haven, CT 06511
203-789-7645

ILLINOIS
Illinois Early Childhood Intervention Clearinghouse
830 S. Spring St. (APD)
Springfield, IL 62704
In IL 800-852-4302 voice, TDD
217-785-1364
Fax 217-524-5339

KENTUCKY
KY-SPIN
Serves Kentucky
2210 Goldsmith Ln. #118 (APD)
Louisville, KY 40218-1038
800-525-SPIN (7746)
502-456-0923

MASSACHUSETTS
Massachusetts Clearinghouse Mutual Support Groups
Univ. of Massachusetts
113 Skinner Hall (APD)
Amherst, MA 01003
413-545-2313

MICHIGAN
Michigan Self-Help Clearinghouse
(Regional)
106 W. Allegan #210 (APD)
Lansing, MI 48933-1706
MI 800-777-5556
Business line 517-484-7373

NEW JERSEY
New Jersey Self-Help Clearinghouse
St. Clares-Riverside Med. Ctr.
25 Pocono Rd. (APD)
Denville, NJ 07834
In NJ 800-FOR-MASH (367-6274)
201-625-9565
TDD 201-625-9035

OREGON
NW Regional Self-Help Clearinghouse
619 S.W. 11th Ave. Rm. 300 (APD)
Portland OR 97205

VIRGINIA
Self-Help Clearinghouse of Greater Washington
Serves Maryland, District of Columbia, Virginia; lists national self-help services
7630 Little River Tpke Ste 206 (APD)
Annandale, VA 22003
703-941-LINK (5465)

WISCONSIN
First Call for Help
17 counties in Wisconsin, Minnesota, Iowa
PO Box 2373 (APD)
La Crosse, WI 54602
WI 800-362-8255
In MN, IA 800-362-8255

Asthma Resources Directory

Clearinghouses

CANADIAN CLEARINGHOUSES
BRITISH COLUMBIA

Family Life Education Council
223 12th Ave. SW (APD)
Calgary, AB T2R 0G9
Canada
403-262-1117

ONTARIO

Canadian Council on Social Development
55 Parkdale Ave. (APD)
PO Box 3505, Station C (APD)
Ottawa, ON K1Y 4G1
Canada
613-728-1865

Community Information Ctr. of the Metropolitan Area
590 Jarvis St. 5th Flr. (APD)
Toronto, ON M4Y 2J4
Canada
416-392-0505

Metropolitan Toronto Self-Help Clearinghouse
40 Orchard View Blvd. Ste. 219 (APD)
Toronto, ON M4R 1B9
416-487-4355

Old Forge Community Resource Center
2730 Curling Ave. (APD)
Ottawa, ON K2B 7J1
613-829-9777

Allergy Products Directory
Copyrighted. Reproduction Prohibited by Law. 1259 El Camino #254, Menlo Park, CA 94025

Asthma Resources Directory
Talking to Your Doctor

Talking to Your Doctor about Asthma

PREPARE FOR YOUR VISIT

Prepare for your visit by writing down your symptoms. Put up a sheet of paper an area of the house that you spend a lot of time.

As something occurs to you, write it down. Think about what you want the doctor to know and write it down. If you have trouble describing the problem, tell the doctor what happens when you try to work, try to go up stairs, try to wash the dishes, try to garden, try to eat a particular food, try to sleep.

Write down questions you want to ask the doctor.

Look through this list. Can you select a chief complaint? Can you point out your major concerns? What makes your symptoms worse or better and when did they start?

Write down questions you want to ask the doctor. It is easy to forget something while you are talking to the doctor and answering questions.

If you are the patient, you may want to arrange to have a friend or family member come with you to the doctor. It helps to have two people listening and remembering.

BRING INFORMATION FOR YOUR DOCTOR'S QUESTIONNAIRE

Questionnaires usually cover your medical history, and may include place of birth, where you have lived, childhood problems, school years, careers. They also include your previous medical problems and hospitalizations, ages or dates, tests, medications, and treatments you have had. Be prepared to answer questions about the health and illnesses of your close relatives.

Carry a list of your immunizations the dates and of your medications.

Carry an emergency information card.

You'll probably need to answer questions about your immunizations and dates. (You should carry this list with you as important information as well as an emergency information card.) Have a list of the medications and dosages that you currently take.

Allergy Products Directory

Copyrighted. Reproduction Prohibited by Law. 1259 El Camino #254, Menlo Park, CA 94025

Asthma Resources Directory

Talking to Your Doctor

Note the name of your current medication, the dosage and how often you take it.

BE PREPARED TO ANSWER QUESTIONS ABOUT YOUR MEDICAL HISTORY

Your doctor will want to know about you.

• What were your previous reactions to drugs, food, pollen, dander, irritants, mold?

• What medications are you currently taking, including vitamins, birth control pills, "natural" medications?

• What kinds of breathing problems have you had?

• Do you experience general shortness of breath, or tightness in the chest?

• Do you cough? What kind of a cough do you have? Is it dry, loose, tight?

• Do you wheeze?

• Do you have other nose or throat problems?

• How long have you had these problems? How old were you went symptoms began?

• How often do you have them?

• Is there a pattern to your symptoms? Do you have them at certain times of the year, certain times of the day or night? Do you have them all the time?

• Does anything make your symptoms worse? Consider exposure to allergens, work exposure, exposure to irritants, medications, foods, exercise, smoke, pets, cold.

AT THE OFFICE

BE PREPARED TO ANSWER QUESTIONS ABOUT YOUR CURRENT PROBLEM

• What asthma medications are you taking now?

• What allergy medications have you taken in the past? Why were they discontinued?

• When you experience the particular symptoms that you are here for, are they related to any specific situation or condition such as cold, exercise, or irritations like fumes, smoke, or odors?

• What makes your symptoms worse or better and when did they start?

Asthma Resources Directory
Talking to Your Doctor

- Have you noticed a difference in your symptoms over time or with a change of location?

- Do animals, feathers, mites, roaches, pollens, or molds bother you? What about aspirin or sulfites?

- Have you had symptoms after taking a particular drug?

- Do you wake up at night?

- How severe are your symptoms?

- Have they changed your life at all?

- Have you been hospitalized recently or had emergency room treatment?

- When are you free of symptoms?

- How often do you use your bronchodilator?

- What other health problems do you have? What medications are you taking for those problems? What dosage do you take and how often?

- Do you smoke? Do others in your home smoke?

- What is your home situation: heating source, age of home, carpeting condition, use of humidifier, pets, exposure to cigarette smoke, smoker?

MEDICATION REACTIONS

If you have ever had a bad reaction from medication, including creams, drops, or oral medications, be sure you keep the name of the medication that caused your problem.

Tell each doctor you see about the reaction so that you will not be prescribed that medication again. Also, be alert to any kind of reaction like slight itching, rash, nausea, or headache when taking a medication and inform your doctor. It may well be that you should not use that medication again.

If you have ever had a bad reaction from medication, be sure to tell each doctor you see.

Discuss other medications that may be related in a pharmacological way to the medication that has given you a problem because you may also react to related medications.

You should know exactly what a medication is supposed to do and how long it should take to work. Ask about side effects. How should you handle a missed dose? How should

Asthma Resources Directory

Talking to Your Doctor

the medication be taken: with meals, on an empty stomach? Is there any food or medication to be avoided while taking this particular medication?

Write down what your doctor says even if you understand it. It is very easy to forget details.

It is very easy to forget details, especially when there are many areas of discussion and a great deal of information is being exchanged.

HOW HAS YOUR PROBLEM AFFECTED YOU?

Have your had serious past reactions? Have you lost days from school? Have you lost days from work? Has this had economic consequences? Have you had to limit your activities? Is your sleep disturbed? Is family life disrupted?

BE SURE YOU UNDERSTAND

Before you leave, be sure you understand what the doctor has said, the reason for any tests to be taken, and the treatment.

1. Know what you must do.

2. Try to review your understanding of the appointment and what has been said.

3. Ask your doctor to correct any misperceptions you may have.

4. Be sure you both agree about what has been said, what treatment is to be followed, what medications are to be used, and what tests are to be taken and why.

5. Ask questions about anything you feel uncertain about or would like to do differently, if possible.

FOLLOW UP

Follow your doctors instructions. They're meant to help you but they won't if you don't follow through. The more you know about your problem, the more control you will have and the better you will handle your situation.

Allergy Products Directory

Copyrighted. Reproduction Prohibited by Law. 1259 El Camino #254, Menlo Park, CA 94025

Asthma Resources Directory

Talking to Your Doctor

AT HOME — BE PREPARED TO CALL

Keep a list of your medications taped near the telephone. The list should include the name of the medication and the doses. Include your doctor's phone numbers and numbers for night and weekend calls.

Keep a list of medications and the doses taped near the telephone.

Include your doctor's phone for day, evening, and weekend calls.

Write down current symptoms and why you are calling. Keep a pad and pen by the phone so that you can write down your doctor's instructions.

If you are calling on a weekend or an evening, your own doctor may not be on duty and his or her colleague may not know you, so it is even more important that you be prepared for your call.

> Sometimes an attack can be averted. If you or your child use a peak flow meter, you will know when to increase medications to lessen the intensity of the attack.
>
> Utilize breathing management and relaxation techniques.
>
> **Don't wait until an attack has progressed to the point that you can tell it is coming.**

If, for some reason your attack is more advanced when you call your doctor, have the following information on hand to save time.

Allowing your doctor to act more efficiently, means that you will have the help you need that much sooner.

If your child is experiencing an attack, tell him or her that you are going to call the doctor. Calm your child and try to remain calm yourself.

Remind your child of breathing and relaxation exercises. If you are experiencing symptoms, try to remain calm. While you are waiting, begin your breathing exercises.

Having information on hand
—Saves time
—Allows your doctor to act more efficiently.
—Gives you the help you need that much sooner.

Asthma Resources Directory
Talking to Your Doctor

CALLING YOUR DOCTOR ✔ CHECK LIST

To call your doctor because of an asthma attack, use this list to help you observe and to organize your thoughts:

Name and age of person

Medications being used_____

Dosages and Times_____

How much medication was taken, how often, how recently.

Describe the symptoms you observe or are experiencing. Symptoms can be different in children and adults.

_____Increased Respiratory Rate (very important)

_____Fast, irregular, or noisy and difficult breathing

_____Wheezing, coughing, or tightness in the chest

_____Pursed lips when breathing out

_____Your peak flow meter reading

_____Grunting
(Area between the ribs looks sunken and concave. Area just below the breast bone is sunken and concave. Stomach moves in and out during breathing. Base of throat, v-notch of collar bone, seems sunken and concave.)

_____Nasal Flaring
(Nostrils are pale blue and move in and out with each breath.)

_____Blueness of the lips, nail beds, or skin

_____Restlessness at night, inability to sleep

_____Need to sit to ease breathing — Hunched posture

_____Unusual paleness

_____Rapid heart beat

_____Vomiting

_____Fatigue

_____Fidgetiness

_____Anxiety or fear

_____Diarrhea

_____ Postnasal drip – excess mucus – what color_____

_____Headache

_____Heartburn

170

Asthma Resources Directory
Talking to Your Doctor

AFTER THE TELEPHONE CALL

> Follow your doctor's instructions. Ask your doctor how long before you should see a response. If you do not see that positive response, call the doctor again. If at all possible, arrange for a time to call back in case there is no improvement. In this way, you won't have to wait for the call to go through again.

10 EMERGENCY SIGNS. SEEK CARE IMMEDIATELY.

1. The wheezing, coughing, or shortness of breath gets worse even 10 minutes after inhaled medication has been used. **You should know how long it takes for your medication or your child's medication to work.**

2. Peak flow rate either drops or remains the same after medication is taken

3. Peak flow rate drops to 50% or less of normal baseline level. This should be discussed in advance with your doctor. You should know the danger zones for peak flow.

4. Breathing is difficult. It is fast, irregular, or noisy. The area between the ribs looks sunken and concave. The area just below the breast bone is sunken and concave.

5. The stomach moves in and out during breathing.

6. Nasal flaring. The nostrils move in and out with each breath.

7. The nostrils are pale blue.

8. Increased respiratory rate.

9. Difficulty walking or talking.

10. Lips or fingernails are grey or blue.

PREPARE FOR THE EMERGENCY ROOM

1. Know your recent steroid medication and dosage.

2. How often do you use your asthma medication? How do you take it?

3. What is your peak flow meter reading when you are well. What is your peak flow meter reading **now**?

4. Have you been hospitalized recently? When? Have you been to the emergency room recently? When?

5. What is your asthma action plan?

171

Allergy Products Directory
Copyrighted. Reproduction Prohibited by Law. 1259 El Camino #254, Menlo Park, CA 94025

Asthma Resources Directory
Camps and Asthma Camps

CHOOSING A CAMP FOR YOUR CHILD

GENERAL CONSIDERATIONS

Look for a camp that generally seems to be a good fit with your child's interests and abilities. Don't send your non-athletic child to a competitive camp and don't send your child who is afraid of large bodies of water to a camp emphasizing lake or ocean swimming and sports. Some camps are purely recreational, some are teaching or special interest camps like tennis, basketball, music, computer, acting, or language. Select on the basis of your child's interest.

Is the camp equipment safe, well-maintained, and age-appropriate?

References are always a good idea and most camps can provide you with telephone numbers of families in your area with whom you may speak. Try to ask your questions neutrally, without hint of the answer you would like. Remember, the families on these lists have had excellent experiences with the camp and want to communicate their enthusiasm to you.

The staff-to-camper ratio can include administrative staff so ask how many counselors sleep in your child's cabin or tent and how many campers sleep in that same cabin or tent. How are counselor's selected? And, if you have selected a special interest camp, ask about the qualifications of counselors.

EVALUATING CAMPS

Camps will need to be evaluated as to how their physical set-up and their camping program meets your child's needs.

Some camps are partaicularly appropriate for children who have physical or mental disabilities. If your child has asthma and disabilities, you may find such a camp suitable. You will want to evaluate the camper population carefully to see if it is a good fit for your child's needs.

One excellent way to evaluate the quality of a camp is to ascertain if it is a member of the American Camping Association. Member camps must meet rigorous standards in administration, programming, personnel, campsite, health care, and camp activities.

Allergy Products Directory

Copyrighted. Reproduction Prohibited by Law. 1259 El Camino #254, Menlo Park, CA 94025

Asthma Resources Directory
Camps and Asthma Camps

You can obtain the American Camping Association's *Guide to Accredited Camps* by writing to:

American Camping Association
Bradford Woods
5000 State Road 67N
Martinsville, IN 46141-7902
800-428-CAMP (2267)

This guide is invaluable for helping you evaluate potential camps for your child.

The guide will help you answer the general kinds of screening questions you will have when choosing a camp for any child such as counselor to camper ratio, kinds of accommodations, etc.

What is the camp's plan of action for reaching emergency care?

Keep in mind the following considerations, when you evaluate a camp in terms of your child's special needs.

✔ Talk to your doctor about the services and facilities your child would need and evaluate each camp based on those needs.

✔ There should be a plan of action for reaching emergency care.

● Is there telephone access? If not, where is the nearest service?

● Consider road conditions. If the road is paved, is it in good condition? Broken pavement means very slow driving. If it is not paved and your climate has summer rain, can the road become muddy and impassable?

Is the nurse's facility on the premises adequate?
Is the off-premise emergency facility adequate?

✔ Consider the emergency facility. Is it adequate? Does it have proper emergency equipment? Is it available twenty-four hours? Who is available to administer care? Is is an RN, a paramedic?

✔ There should be access to medical care on the premises. Consider the nurse's facility.

● Does the cabin have a quiet room.

● Are the campers' medications kept under lock and key, clearly identified, and with instructions for their use?

173

Asthma Resources Directory
Camps and Asthma Camps

● Is the room clean and dust-free? Is it air conditioned or filtered?

✔ Is the camp willing to handle food allergies? Will the camp allow you to store any special food your child may need and allow your child access to them? A Jewish camp that keeps kosher will understand how to manage your child's milk-elimination diet.

✔ What kinds of trees are in the area? Are there trees that your child is allergic to or is the pollen count low for the pollen that trigger your child's asthma or allergic rhinitis? What kinds of pollen can the winds bring toward the camping area?

✔ As far as climate and altitutde, would your child be better off in a forest location, a beach area, a desert location or in a city dormitory?

A Jewish camp that keeps kosher will understand how to manage your child's milk-elimination diet or lactose intolerance.

✔ Camps that specialize in sports or specific activities may be advantageous to your child. For example, if your child has exercise-induced bronchospasm, swimming camps are a good idea If animals or hayrides are your child's potential triggers, consider a watersports camp instead. If your child has a pollen problem, consider a talent camp in the city or a beach camp. If your child has a particular talent or interest, consider a drama, computer, language or singing camp.

✔ The grounds should be smoke-free and safe for free activities as well as organized ones.

✔ Are there comfortable places to rest?

✔ How convenient are drinking fountains?

✔ Will your child live in a tent, a cabin, a dorm? Does the tent smell of mildew? Is the cabin (and mattress) clean? Bring a mattress and pillow encasing or bring your child's own pillow with cover from home. Is the dorm air conditioned? Is there a mildew odor on the furniture?

TALKING WITH CAMP PERSONNEL

The camp should be informed in advance and in writing of all of your child's special needs so that there are no unpleasant surprises when you arrive. Bring several copies of your letter with you.

Asthma Resources Directory
Camps and Asthma Camps

Try to arrive early so that you can be sure that your child's counselor has been informed. If the counselor has not been informed, you will then have the time to go over important information and leave a copy of the letter. Discuss current medication, symptoms, storage for foods, and any last minute questions.

Also talk to the nurse, the doctor, if there is one, and the camp director. You will want to remind everyone of the arrangements agreed upon and familiarize your child with the camp's layout.

✔ Show your child the way to the nurse's cabin and make introductions.

Provide extra medications and food in case of loss, breakage, or a need for increased medication.

Be sure everything is clearly labeled with your child's name and that instructions for medications are clear.

✔ Explain to the counselor your child's health needs. Be specific. Mention remaining upwind from campfires or not being kept out of group activities. Ask if medications (inhalers) can be available. Ask about camp policy for peak flow meters. If the child needs to be brought to the nurse for medications or only reminded, arrangements should be made at this time.

✔ Provide the nurse with your doctor's medical plan for your child's asthma. This should include medication schedule and dosage.

✔ Provide camp leaders with adequate emergency referrals in case you are not immediately available. Have several telephone numbers available as well as an emergency physician resource.

If food allergies are a consideration, be sure your child's special foods are labeled with your child's name and name and number.

✔ Provide extra medications and food in case of loss, breakage, or a need for increased medication. Be sure everything is clearly labeled with your child's name and that instructions for medications are clear. If food allergies are a consideration, now is the time to talk to the camp cook and store any special foods you may have brought. Be sure the foods are labeled with your child's name and with your name and telephone number.

Asthma Resources Directory

Camps and Asthma Camps

✔ If it is not possible for you to be at the camp, be sure to call and speak with everyone involved. Visit at the first opportunity in order to follow-up.

EVALUATING ASTHMA REHABILITATION PROGRAMS AND ASTHMA CAMPS

With the passage of the Americans with Disabilities Act, camps are now required to serve those with disabilities. Some, of course, are able to handle some disabilities better than others. Your family needs to decide if it is better for your child to be in a specialized camp or to be part of a wide group, most of whom will have no health problems or disabilities. If the need to be educated in asthma procedures is paramount, choose an asthma camp.

An excellent source of information is *Summer Camps for Children with Asthma* from the American Lung Association 1829 Portland Ave., Minneapolis, MN 55404-1898, 612-871-7332.

WHAT TO LOOK FOR IN AN ASTHMA REHABILITATION PROGRAM

✔ CHECK LIST

The purpose of sending your child to an asthma camp is to educate and to give your child an understanding of the problem and its treatment, as well as to provide a pleasurable camping experience. The end goal is to allow the child to enjoy a other types of camping experiences.

The program should address. . .

• Breathing Techniques

• Correct Use of Inhaler

• Importance of Peak Flow Monitoring and how to use one

• Common side effects of medication and how to control them

• Stress Management: how to use breathing techniques and other relaxation techniques to modify stress

• Signs of Trouble: how to recognize the need for self-medication and how to evaluate its effectiveness; when to call the doctor; how to manage until help is available

Asthma Resources Directory
Camps and Asthma Camps

- Monitoring Progress: how to use a peak flow meter; detecting impending trouble before wheezing begins or other symptoms occur

- Exercise: how to determine proper heart rate; exercises best suited to you; warming up, cooling down

- Triggers: recognizing the causes of your attacks: locating and eliminating triggers in the home

- controlling the environment; avoiding or reducing the effects of triggers

- Travel: how to plan for safe travel; medications to take; taking medications while passing through time zones; checking on climate conditions, altitude, smoke-free accommodations; what to do if you become ill away from home

- The program should be organized so that taking of medication has minimal interference with activities

- Treatments should be timely and campers should not wait about. Know who supervises treatments and medications

- Is there a self-medication program that helps develop independence and if so, how is it monitored to assure compliance?

- What is the procedure for peak flow meter readings?

- Who assess the campers and how often?

- What is the procedure for episodes of night wheezing or coughing?

EVALUATING ASTHMA CAMP PROGRAMS

Why should your child go to an asthma camp? An asthma camp teaches your child, in a safe environment, that he or she can function even with asthma. A good program addresses independence, self-image, and provides factual information about asthma and lungs. Some programs are for children only, others involve parents.

In an asthma camp, children have a wonderful opportunity to enjoy themselves and to gain control over their environments.

Children should go to camp to have fun. They may learn physical skills and social skills, but they should also have fun. In an asthma camp, children have a wonderful opportunity to enjoy themselves and to gain control over their environments. A good asthma camp program can

177

Asthma Resources Directory

Camps and Asthma Camps

teach your child to understand, control, and live with asthma, gain confidence and self-esteem, and learn about allergy treatment under professional guidance.

A GOOD ASTHMA CAMP PROGRAM SHOULD TEACH YOUR CHILD

✔ CHECK LIST

- To recognize what bring on an attack for him or her.

- To locate and eliminate triggers at home, to control the environment as much as possible.

- To avoid or reduce the effect of triggers.

- The signs of trouble; how to recognize the need for self-medication; when to call the doctor; how to manage until help is available.

- Breathing techniques.

- To use an inhaler properly.

- About common medication side effects and how to control them.

- To use a peak flow meter to monitor progress and avert problems before wheezing or other symptoms occur.

- To exercise safely; to determine proper heart rate; to select the exercises best suited to the child's condition; how to warm up; how to cool down

- To avoid cigarette smoke and smoking and how to handle social pressures related to smoking.

The advantages of sending your child to an asthma camp are many. Your child will:

1. Work toward physical fitness in a safe environment

2. See that others attain goals

3. Gain confidence in his or her ability to handle asthma

4. Gain factual information about asthma

EVALUATE THE PHYSICAL FACILITY
✔ CHECK LIST

You will want to evaluate the physical set-up of the asthma camp. Some of the items you will want to consider are. . .

• Is the doctor full time? What is his or her specialty?

• Is a nurse available full time?

• How can the doctor or nurse be reached when he or she is not in the infirmary?

• Are there respiratory therapists on staff?

• Will your child carry his or her own medications (inhaler)?

• Will your child be able to use his or her own peak flow meter?

• Is the infirmary fully equipped with appropriate medications and equipment for asthma and for non-asthma problems? Is there an isolation room? Will medication be given according to the schedule you specify? Is it available twenty-four hours?

• Is there convenient and rapid access to a nearby medical center or hospital, paramedics or fire house? How far away is the facility? Are emergency procedures and telephone numbers immediately accessible? Are roads paved for rapid transportation? If you live in a climate with summer rain, is the road paved or will it become muddy and impassable in the rain?

• If there are outings away from the camp facility or overnights, is emergency equipment taken by someone who is qualified to handle it?

• What kinds of trees are in the area? Are there trees that your child is allergic to or is the pollen count low for the pollen that triggers your child's asthma? Can the prevailing winds carry problem-causing pollen from more distant areas? Would your child be better off in a forest location, beach area, desert location or in a city dormitory?

• The grounds should be smoke-free and safe

• What kind of insurance coverage does the camp have?

• If your child has food allergy problems, will the camp provide substitutes or will it allow you to bring and store the special foods your child will need?

Asthma Resources Directory
Camps and Asthma Camps

EVALUATE THE GOALS OF THE PROGRAM
✔ CHECK LIST

You will also want to evaluate the program of the asthma camp. You want to know that the program will. . .

• Educate your child in the management of asthma. Teach your child to identify and respond to early warning signals

• Teach your child to identify and avoid personal triggers

• Teach your child relaxation techniques and breathing techniques

• Teach your child coping skills: psychosocial aspects; how to talk with friends about asthma

• Show your child how to use an inhaler or an inhaler with spacer properly and a peak flow meter

Ask for a summary of your child's experiences at the camp. You'll want to know about health and social activities and how the educational activities were assessed

EVALUATE YOUR CHILD'S EXPERIENCE
✔ CHECK LIST

When trying to evaluate how your child benefited from asthma camp, you can consider the following. . .

• Are you seeing emotional changes? Is your child more confident? Have peer relationships improved?

• Is your child using less medication or using medication earlier or more effectively?

• Are there fewer emergency room visits?

• Are there fewer days lost from school or normal activities?

DEVELOP A TRAVEL PLAN

To prepare for an overnight camp, you also need to develop a travel plan for your child. You'll want to discuss with your doctor, the adults in charge, and your child the following. . .

• What medications to take

• How to take medications while traveling through time zones

Allergy Products Directory

Copyrighted. Reproduction Prohibited by Law. 1259 El Camino #254,Menlo Park, CA 94025

Asthma Resources Directory
Camps and Asthma Camps

- Are the accommodations smoke-free?

- What can be done if your child becomes ill while traveling

Our special thanks to Penny Gottier-Fena, American Lung Assn. of Minneapolis for her help with the listing of summer camps here.

HELP US TO HELP YOU

When writing to the companies and organizations listed here, be sure to use the initials (APD) as part of the address and tell them you saw them listed in *Allergy Products Directory.*

If you call, be sure to tell them you found them in *Allergy Products Directory.*

This is important to you because:

- Lets the company know that its listings have helped you.

- Encourages the company to keep *Allergy Products Directory* informed of its new products so that we can keep you informed.

- Enables us to keep our listings accurate and up-to-date for you on the latest products, services, and innovations.

- Enables us to keep the Directory price low for you.

Thank you for your help.

Allergy Products Directory
Copyrighted. Reproduction Prohibited by Law. 1259 El Camino #254, Menlo Park, CA 94025

Asthma Resources Directory
Asthma Camps

ASTHMA CAMPS

Not all camps will be available each year. Please call the location nearest you for current information or call the American Lung Association at 800-LUNG-USA (586-4872) or the Asthma and Allergy Foundation of America 202-466-7643

The camps listed here have not been inspected or recommended, guaranteed, or warranteed in any way either as to the operation of the camp or the program, or any of the individuals conducting the program or designing it.

ALASKA

Champ Camp
American Lung Assn./Alaska
1057 W. Fireweed Ln. (APD)
Anchorage, AK 99503
907-276-5864

ARKANSAS

Camp Aldersgate
2000 Aldersgate Rd. (APD)
Little Rock, AR 72205
501-225-1444
ACA accredited

ARIZONA

Not-A-Wheeze
Arizona Lung Asssn.
102 W. McDowell Rd. (APD)
Phoenix, AZ 85003
602-258-7505

CALIFORNIA

AAFA Asthma Camp
Asthma & Allergy Foundation/Los Angeles
5225 Wilshire Blvd. #705 (APD)
Los Angeles, CA 90036
213-937-90036

ALA Camp
American Lung Association/Santa Cruz/San Luis Obispo
140 Central Ave. (APD)
Salinas, CA 93901

408-757-5864

Asthma Camp
Long Beach Lung Assn.
CSU Dept. of PE
1250 Bellflower Blvd. (APD)
Long Beach, CA 90840
310-985-4077
310-985-7969

Asthma Education Day Camp
Various locations
American Lung Assn./Redwood Empire
PO Box 1482 (APD)
Santa Rosa, CA 95402-1482
707-527-5864

Asthma Education Family Camp
Various locations
American Lung Assn./Redwood Empire
PO Box 1482 (APD)
Santa Rosa, CA 95402-1482
707-527-5864

Breathe Easy Day Camp
American Lung Assn./Alameda County
295 27th St. (APD)
Oakland, CA 94563
510-893-5474

Camp Discovery
American Lung Association/Central California
234 N. Broadway (APD)
Fresno, CA 943701
209-266-5864

Asthma Resources Directory

Asthma Camps

Camp Sierra
American Lung Assn./Central
California
234 N. Broadway (APD)
Fresno, CA 93701
209-266-5864

Camp Superkids
Salilnas Valley Memorial Hospital
Respiratory Care Dept.
450 E. Romie Ln. (APD)
Salinas, CA 93901
408-757-4333 Exts. 1652, 1782, 1436

Camp Superstuff
American Lung Assn./Central
California
PO Box 11187 (APD)
Fresno, CA 93772-1187
209-266-5864

Camp Superstuff
American Lung Assn./Francisco
562 Mission St. (APD)
San Francisco, CA 94105
415-543-4410

Camp Superstuff
American Lung Assn./Santa Clara,
San Benito
1469 Park Ave. (APD)
San Jose, CA 95126
408-998-5864 (998-LUNG)

Camp Superstuff
American Lung Assn./Superior
California
2723 Cohasset Rd. #A (APD)
Chico, CA 95926-0977
916-345-5864

Camp Wheeze
American Lung Assn.
Ask for Joann Blessing-Moore, MD
530 El Camino Real (APD)
Burlingame, CA 94010
415-343-3978

Camp Wheeze
American Lung Assn./San Mateo

2250 Palm Ave. (APD)
San Mateo, CA 94403-1860
415-349-1111

Champ Camp
American Lung Assn./Contra Costa,
Solano
105 Astrid Dr. (APD)
Pleasant Hill, CA 94523-4399
415-935-0472

Children's Asthma Camp
American Lung Assn./Los Angeles
County
5858 Wilshire Blvd. #300 (APD)
PO Box 36926 (APD)
Los Angeles, CA 90036-0926
213-935-5864

SCAMP Camp
American Lung Assn./Imperial
Counties
2750 Fourth Ave. (APD)
PO Box 3879 (APD)
San Diego, CA 92103
619-297-3901

Scamp Camp
American Lung Assn./Inland
Counties- San Bernardino, Inyo, Mono
371 W. 14th St. (APD)
San Bernardino, CA 92405
909-884-5864

Scamp Camp
American Lung Assn./Orange County
1570 E. 17th St. (APD)
Santa Ana, CA 92701
714-835-LUNG (835-5864)

SCAMP Camp
American Lung Assn./San Diego,
Imperial Counties
2750 Fourth Ave. (APD)
San Diego, CA 92103
619-297-3901

Asthma Resources Directory

Asthma Camps

COLORADO

Champ Camp
American Lung Assn./Colorado
National Jewish Center for
Immunology/Respiratory Medicine
1600 Race St. (APD)
Denver, CO 80206-1198
800-LUNG-USA (586-4872)
303-388-4327

CONNECTICUT

Camp Treasure Chest
American Lung Assn./Connecticut
45 Ash St. (APD)
E. Hartford, CT 06108
203-289-5401

DISTRICT OF COLUMBIA

Camp Happy Lungs
American Lung Asson./District of
Columbia
475 H St. N.W. (APD)
Washington, DC 20001
202-682-5864

FLORIDA

Camp Superstuff
American Lung Assn./Dade-Monroe,
Inc.
830 Brickell Plaza (APD)
Miami, FL 33131-3996
800-524-8010

Sunshine Station
American Lung Asson./Florida
PO Box 8127 (APD)
Jacksonville, FL 32239-8127
904-743-2933

GEORGIA

Asthma Day Camp
American Lung Assn./Georgia, W.
Central Branch

4570 Reese Rd. (APD)
Columbus, GA 31907
706-569-1098

Camp Breathe Easy
American Lung Assn./Atlanta
723 Piedmont Ave. N.E. (APD)
Atlanta, GA 30365-0701
404-872-9653

Camp Breathe Easy
American Lung Assn./Georgia
2452 Spring Rd. (APD)
Smyrna, GA 30080
404-434-5864

Superstuff Summer
American Lung Association/Georgia,
S.W. Branch
1104 B. 3rd. Ave. (APD)
PO Box 70174 (APD)
Albany, GA 31707
912-435-3626

HAWAII

Hawaii Asthma Camp
Young Buddhist Assn. of Honolulu
1710 Pali Highway (APD)
Honolulu, HI 96813

Kokua Ma Kuki
American Lung Assn./Hawaii
245 N. Kukui St. (APD)
Honolulu, HI 96817
808-537-5966

IOWA

Camp Superkids
American Lung Assn./Iowa
1025 Ashworth Rd. #410 (APD)
W. Des Moines, IA 50265-6600
515-224-0800

Asthma Resources Directory

Asthma Camps

ILLINOIS

Camp ACTION
American Lung Assn./Metropolitan
Chicago
1440 W. Washington Blvd. (APD)
Chicago, IL 60607-1878
312-243-2000

Camp Superkids
American Lung Assn./Illinois
#1 Christmas Seal Dr. (APD)
PO Box 2576 (APD)
Springfield, IL 62708
217-528-3441

INDIANA

Camp Superkids Resident Camp
American Lung Assn./Northern
Indiana
319 S. Main St. (APD)
South Bend, IN 46601
219-287-2321

Camp Superkids
American Lung Assn./Indiana
9410 Priority Way W. (APD)
Indianapolis, IN 46240
317-573-3900

Camp Superkids
American Lung Assn./Northern
Indiana
319 S. Main St. (APD)
South Bend, IN 46601
219-287-2321

Camp Superkids
American Lung Assn./Northwest
Indiana
6685 Broadway (APD)
Merrillville, IN 46410
219-769-4264

Camp Superkids
American Lung Assn./Southwest
Indiana
7 E. Columbia St. (APD)
PO Box 4136 (APD)

Evansville, IN 47711
812-422-3402

KANSAS

Camp Superbreathers
American Lung Assn.
1107 Parklane Office Park #224 (APD)
Wichita, KS 67207
316-687-3888

KENTUCKY

Camp Superkids
American Lung Assn./Kentucky
PO Box 969 (APD)
Louisville, KY 40201
502-363-2652

LOUISIANA

Camp Azzie
Opelousas General Hospital
PO Box 1208 (APD)
Opelousas, LA 70570
318-948-5186
318-948-3011 Ext. 598

MASSACHUSETTS

Camp Chest Nut
American Lung Assn./Massachusetts
1505 Commonwealth Ave. (APD)
Brighton, MA 2135
617-787-LUNG (5864)

MARYLAND

Camp Breathe Easy
American Lung Assn./Maryland
251 E. Antietam St. (APD)
Hagerstown, MD 21740
301-790-8192

Camp Breathe Easy
Franklin Square Hospital Ctr.
9000 Franklin Sq. Dr. (APD)
Baltimore, MD 21237

185

Asthma Resources Directory

Asthma Camps

410-682-7012

Camp Superkids
American Lung Assn./Maryland
1840 York Rd., #K-M (APD)
Timonium, MD 21093-5156
410-560-2120

MAINE

Camp Opportunity
American Lung Assn./Maine
128 Sewall St. (APD)
Augusta, ME 04330
207-622-6394

MICHIGAN

Camp Michi-Mac
American Lung Assn./Michigan
Asthma & Allergy Foundation of
America
607 Grove St. (APD)
Hudson, MI 49247
517-448-8543

Camp Sun Deer
American Lung Assn./Southeast
Michigan
18860 W. Ten Mile Rd. (APD)
Southfield, MI 48075
810-559-5100

MINNESOTA

Camp Superkids
American Lung Assn./Hennepin
American Lung Assn./Minnesota
1829 Portland Ave. (APD)
Minneaplis, MN 55404-1898
612-871-7332

Camp We No Wheeze North
American Lung Assn./Minnesota
424 W. Superior St. #203 (APD)
Duluth, MN 55802
218-726-4721

MISSOURI

Asthma Camp of Western Missouri
American Lung Assn./W. Missouri
2401 Gillham (APD)
Kansas City, MO 64108
816-234-3097

Camp Superkids
American Lung Assn./E. Missouri
1118 Hampton Ave. (APD)
St. Louis, MO 63139-3196
314-645-5505

MONTANA

Camp Huff 'n Puff
American Lung Assn./Montana
825 Helena Ave. (APD)
Helena, MT 59601
406-442-6556

NORTH CAROLINA

Camp Challenge
American Lung Assn./North Carolina
3901 Baarrett Dr. #313 (APD)
Raleigh, NC 27609
919-782-2888

Camp Challenge
American Lung Assn./North Carolina
3901 Barrett Dr. #313 (APD)
Raleigh, NC 27609
919-782-2888

Camp Mountain Air
American Lung Assn./North Carolina
390 S. French Broad Rd. (APD)
Asheville, NC 28801
704-254-5366

NORTH DAKOTA

Dakota Superkids Asthma Camp
American Lung Assn./North Carolina
212 N. 2nd St. (APD)
PO Box 5004 (APD)

Asthma Resources Directory

Asthma Camps

Bismarck, ND 58502-5004
800-252-6325
701-223-5613

NEBRASKA

Camp Superkids
American Lung Assn./Nebraska
7101 Newport Ave. #303 (APD)
Omaha, NE 68152
402-572-3030

NEW HAMPSHIRE

Camp Superkids
American Lung Assn./New Hampshire
456 Beech St. (APD)
PO Box 1014 (APD)
Manchester, NH 03105
603-669-2411

NEW JERSEY

Camp Superkids
American Lung Assn./New Jersey
1600 Rt. 22 E. (APD)
Union, NJ 07083-3407
908-687-9340

NEW MEXICO

Stephen Lopez Camp for Children with Asthma
American Lung Assn./New Mexico
216 Truman N.E. (APD)
Albuquerque, NM 87108
505-265-0732

NEVADA

Camp Superkids
American Lung Assn./Nevada
6119 Ridgeview Ct. (APD)
Reno, NV 89509
702-825-5864

Camp Superkids
American Lung Assn./Nevada
4100 Boulder Hwy. #D (APD)
Las Vegas, NV 89121
702-454-2500

NEW YORK

Camp Superkids Day Camp
American Lung Assn./Queens
112-25 Queens Blvd. (APD)
Forest Hills, NY 11375
718-263-5656

Camp Superkids Sleepaway
American Lung Assn./Queens
112-25 Queens Blvd. (APD)
Forest Hills, NY 11375
718-263-5656

Camp Superkids
American Lung Assn./Mid-New York
1249 Front St. #105 (APD)
Binghamton, NY 13905
607-772-8422

St. James Mercy Hospital Annual Asthma Camp
St. James Mercy Hospital
411 Canisteo St. (APD)
Hornell, NY 14843
607-324-3900 Ext. 3358

Superkids at Camp Chingachgook
American Lung Assn./N.E. New York
8 Mountainview Ave. (APD)
Albany, NY 12205
518-459-4197

OHIO

Camp Superkids at Camp Timberlane
American Lung Assn./Ohio, South Shore Branch
226 State Rt. 61 E. (APD)
Norwalk, OH 44857
419-663-LUNG (5864)

187

Asthma Resources Directory

Asthma Camps

Camp Superkids
American Lung Assn./S.W.Ohio
11135 Kenwood Rd. (APD)
Cincinnati, OH 45242
513-985-3990

Camp Superkids
American Lung Assn./N.W. Ohio
4759 Violet Rd. (APD)
Toledo, OH 43623
419-471-0024

Camp Superkids
American Lung Assn./N.E. Ohio
2703 Mahoning Ave. #207 (APD)
Youngstown, OH 44509
216-792-1215

Camp Superkids
American Lung Assn./OH Greater
Dayton Area
PO Box 5759 (APD)
Dayton, OH 45405
513-277-3300

OKLAHOMA

Camp Breathe Easy
American Lung Assn./Oklahoma
2442 N. Walnut (APD)
PO Box 53303 (APD)
Oklahoma City, OK 73152-3303
405-524-8471

Ella Davis Crewson Asthma Control Camp
American Lung Assn./Green County
2805 E. Skelly Dr. #806 (APD)
Tulsa, OK 74105
918-747-3441

OREGON

Camp Christmas Seal
American Lung Assn./Oregon
1776 S.W. Madison St. (APD)
Portland, OR 97205-1798
503-224-5145

PENNSYLVANIA

Breathe E-Z
American Lung Assn./Western
Pennsylvania
Various locations
PO Box 100 (APD)
Warrendale, PA 15086
In PA: 800-220-1990
412-772-1750

Camp Breathe Easy
American Lung Assn./Central
Pennsylvania
PO Box 1632 (APD)
Harrisburg, PA 17105-1632
717-234-5991

Camp Huff 'n Puff
American Lung Assn./Western
Pennsylvania
PO Box 100 (APD)
Warrendale, PA 15086
In PA: 800-220-1990
412-772-1750

Camp Puff-n-Stuff
American Lung Assn./Central
Pennsylvania
1201 Grampian Blvd. #1C (APD)
Wiliamsport, PA 17701
717-326-8270

Camp SuperKids
American Lung Assn./Central
Pennsylvania
205 E. Beaver Ave. (APD)
State College, PA 16801
814-234-8037

Camp Superstuff
American Lung Assn./N.W.
Pennsylvania
352 W. 8th St. (APD)
Erie, PA 16502
814-454-0109

Upward Bound Asthma Camp
American Lung Assn./N.E.
Pennsylvania

Asthma Resources Directory

Asthma Camps

206 E. Brown St. (APD)
E. Stroudsburg, PA 18301
717-476-3552

SOUTH CAROLINA

Camp Puff 'n Stuff
American Lung Assn./South Caroalina
1941 Savage Rd. #200A (APD)
Charleston, SC 29407
803-556-8451

SOUTH DAKOTA

McKennan Airway Care "MAC" Camp
McKennan Hospital
Children's Miracle Network
YMCA
Various locations
800 E. 21st. St. (APD)
Sioux Falls, SD 57117-5045
In SD: 800-331-2273
800-223-1558

TENNESSEE

Camp Wezbegon East
American Lung Assn./Tennessee
1808 W. End Ave. #514
Nashville, TN 37203
800-432-LUNG (5864)
615-329-1151

Camp Wezbegon West
American Lung Assn./Tennessee
1808 W. End Ave. #514
Nashville, TN 37203
800-432-LUNG (5864)
615-329-1151

TEXAS

Camp Broncho
American Lung Assn./Texas
4502 Centerview Dr. #116 (APD)
San Antonio, TX 78228
210-734-5864

Jeff A. Green Asthma Camp
American Lung Assn./Dallas-N.E.
7616 LBJ Freeway, #100 (APD)
Dallas, TX 75251
214-239-5864

UTAH

Camp Wyatt
American Lung Assn./Utah
1930 S. 1100 E. (APD)
Salt Lake City, UT 84106
801-484-4456

VIRGINIA

Camp Superkids
American Lung Assn./Virginia
311 South Blvd. (APD)
Richmond, VA 23220
800-345-LUNG (5864)
804-355-3295

Camp Superkids
American Lung Assn./Virginia, S.W.
PO Box 1249 (APD)
Abingdon, VA 24210
703-628-1277

Camp Superkids
American Lung Assn./Virginia,
Central, Roanoke
6318 Peters Creek Rd. NW (APD)
Roanoke, VA 24019
703-362-5864

Camp Superstuff
American Lung Association/Virginia,
S.E. Area
5349 E. Princess Anne Rd. (APD)
Norfolk, VA 23502
804-855-3059

New River Valley Asthma Day Camp for Youth
Radford Community Hospital
700 Randolph St. (APD)
Radford, VA 24141
703-731-2645

Asthma Resources Directory

Asthma Camps

WASHINGTON

Asthma Camp at Camp Sealth
American Lung Assn./Washington
2203 N. 30th St. (APD)
Tacoma, WA 98403
206-272-8777

Camp Breathe Easy
American Lung Assn./Washington
901 Summitview Ave. #241 (APD)
Yakima, WA 98902
509-248-4384

Camp CHAMP
American Lung Assn./Washington
N. 1322 Ash (APD)
Spokane, WA 99201
800-732-9339
509-325-6516

Children's Orthopedic Hospital Camp
Children's Orthopedic Hospital
4800 Sandpoint Way N.E.
Seattle, WA 98105
206-634-5423

WISCONSIN

Camp WIDIDAS
American Lung Assn./Wisconsin
150 S. Sunnyslope Rd. #105 (APD)
Brookfield, WI 53005
414-782-7833

Allergy Products Directory
Copyrighted. Reproduction Prohibited by Law. 1259 El Camino #254, Menlo Park, CA 94025

Asthma Resources Directory

Special Services

SPECIAL SERVICES

CONSULTING SERVICES

Allergy/Asthma DATASearch

American Allergy Assn. will search its database of thousands of listings for information on allergy, asthma, food allergy products, services, resources and where to find help. Donation requested.
AllergyAid@aol.com

Allergy Relief Shop Consulting Services

Phone consultation, product recommendation; on-site consultation and recommendations; considers mold, remodeling, duct work, heating systems, dust

Cotton mattresses in custom sizes; cotton futons in varying sizes
Available from:
Allergy Relief Shop,™Inc.
3371 Whittle Springs Rd. (APD)
Knoxville, TN 37917
Orders 800-626-2810
Questions 615-522-2795

Camp Advisory Service

If you need a camp in a certain geographical area because of your child's allergy or asthma constraints, this service will let you know which camps are in that area and what they specialize in: music, sports, computer, etc.
Available from:
Camp Advisory Service
501 E. Boston Post Rd. (APD)
Mamaroneck, NY 10543
212-696-0499

Dietitian Referral in Spanish

Available from:
American Dietetic Assn.
216 W. Jackson Blvd. #800 (APD)
Chicago, IL 60606-6995
312-899-0040

Fax 312-899-1979

Footwear Industries of America

If you have an unusual shoe problem, this organization may be of help
Footwear Industries of America
1420 K St. NW, Ste. 600 (APD)
Washington, DC 20005-2505
202-789-1420
Fax 202-789-4058

Imperial Adhesives & Chemicals

If you have an unusual shoe problem relating to adhesives, this company may be of help
Imperial Adhesives & Chemicals
6315 Wiehe Rd. (APD)
Cincinnati, OH 45237-4277
800-365-1301
513-351-1300
Fax 513-351 1994

Insurance Liaison

800-423-8891 Ext. 1571
Discusses insurance coverage for clinic programs with your insurance carrier if there is a question about coverage
Available from:
National Jewish Center for Immunology
and Respiratory Medicine
1400 Jackson at ColFax (APD)
Denver, CO 80206-2762
800-222-LUNG (5864)
In CO 303-355-LUNG (5864)
303-398-1907

Product Specialist

800-537-8484
Discusses product function and appropriateness for your need (The Protector insect trap)

Asthma Resources Directory

Special Services

United Shoe Machinery

If you have an unusual shoe problem relating to adhesives, this company may be of help
United Shoe Machinery Corp.
400 Research Dr. (APD)
Wilmington, MA 01887-1055
508-657-4700
Fax 508-658-7459

HOUSEHOLD SERVICES

ALK Indoor Allergen Analysis

Test measures cat and mice allergen levels in dust samples from living or working environment; repeat measurements monitor effectiveness.
Orders 800-326-9181 Ext. 222
Available from:
ALK Indoor Allergen Analysis
PO Box 200 (APD)
Spring Mills, PA 16875-9988
814-422-8165

Allergy Clean Environments

Custom size encasings for bedding; comforter encasings
Available from:
Allergy Clean Environments
501 Station Ave. (APD)
Haddon Heights, NJ 08035
800-882-4110
In NJ 609-546-1101
Fax 609-546-1466
URL:
http:\\WWW.infomall.com\allergy.html

Allergy Relief Products Ltd.

Dust-proof encasings made to size for cots, futons, cushions, bunkbeds
Available from:
Allergy Relief Products, Ltd.
39 Spring Crescent (APD)
Southampton SO2 1FZ
England
44-0703-586709
Fax 44-0703-676226

Allergy Relief Products, Ltd.

Custom size dust-proof mattress, pillow, duvet, encasings
Available from:
Allergy Relief Products
9 Renata Ct. (APD)
Dundas, ON L9H 6X1
Canada
905-628-5324 ?416
Fax 416-628-1734

Dona Designs

Custom size futons
Available from:
Dona Designs
1611 Bent Tree St. (APD)
Seagoville, TX 75159
214-287-7834
Don & Dona Shrier

Dust Analysis Test

Separate tests for your house dust; collector and instructions provided; test for dust mite allergen, cockroach, cat, cat allergen; mold spore count
Available from:
Allergy-Asthma Shopper™
PO Box 239 (APD)
Fate, TX 75132
800-447-1100
Fax 903-883-4513

Mold Test Plate

Kit allows you to collect samples at home in a U.S. Postal Service approved sample collection and shipping container with label; sample is mailed to EPA certified labaoratory for analysis and report
Available from:
Allergy Resources
Mail: PO Box 888 (APD)
UPS: 264 Brookridge Ave. (APD)
Palmer Lake, CO 80133
Orders 800-USE-FLAX (873-3529)
Company plans to move; use 800 #

Asthma Resources Directory

Special Services

Touch of Class

Custom size envelopes made from sheets protect comforters; act as duvets
Available from:
Touch of Class
1905 N. Van Buren St. (APD)
Huntingburg, IN 47542-9595
800-457-7456
Fax 812-683-5921

AIR DUCT CLEANING SERVICES

Absolute Air Duct Cleaning

Cleans dust, molds, bacteria from central air conditioning systems and ventillation systems, dryer vents, building intakes; residential, commercial, industrial. Serves Dade, Broward, and Palm Beach counties in Florida
Available from:
Absolute Environmental's Allergy Store
2615 S. University Dr. (APD)
Davie, FL 33328
Nationwide 800-771-ACHOO (2246)
In FL 800-329-3773
Broward 305-472-3773
Fax 305-474-0133

Air Doctors, Inc.

Cleans bacteria and fungi from ducts and vents of heating, ventilating, and air conditioning systems; residential, commercial, industrial
Available from:
Air Doctors, Inc.
3632 Meadow Ln. (APD)
Jackson, MS 39212
PO Box 7147 (APD)
Jackson, MS 39282-7147
601-371-8928
Fax 601-373-2623

Clean Air Services

Cleans dust, molds, bacteria from central air conditioning systems and ventillation systems

Available from:
Clean Air Services
2402 Elm St. (APD)
Allentown, PA 18104
215-435-4355
Fax 215-435-4295

FILTER SERVICES

3M Company

PO Box 33275 (APD)
St. Paul, MN 55133-3275
3M Center Bldg.(APD)
St. Paul, MN 55144-1000
Medical information 800-328-0255
Medical information local 612-736-4930
Customer service 800-423-5197
Outside CA 800-423-5146
In CA 818-341-1300

AAir Purification Systems

7340 Trade St. #C (APD)
San Diego, CA 92121-2457
800-776-6746
619-578-2825
Fax 619-578-3762

Absolute Environmental's Allergy Store

2615 S. University Dr. (APD)
Davie, FL 33328
800-771-ACHOO (2246) nationwide
In FL 800-329-3773
Broward 305-472-3773
Fax 305-474-0133

Aller-Guard,® Inc.

Southgate Office Park
1645 S.W. 41st St. (APD)
Topeka, KS 66609-1250
800-234-0816
913-267-9333
Fax 913-267-0072

Allergy Control Products, Inc.

96 Danbury Rd. (APD)
PO Box 793 (APD)
Ridgefield, CT 06877

193

Asthma Resources Directory

Special Services

800-422-DUST (3878)
203-438-9580
Fax 203-431-8963

Allergy Supply Co., Inc. The
11994 Star Court (APD)
Herndon, VA 22071
800-323-6744
Metropolitan DC 703-391-2011
Fax 703-391-2014
BBS 703-521-0638

Appliance Sales & Service Co.
655 Mission St. (APD)
San Francisco, CA 94105
800-424-6783
In 415 area call 415-362-7195

DeVilbiss
Sunrise Medical/DeVilbiss, Inc.
PO Box 635 (APD)
Somerset, PA 15501-0635
800-DeV-1988 (338-1988)
814-443-4881
Fax 800-345-2202
In Canada 705-728-5522

Environtrol® Corp.
PO Box 31313 (APD)
St. Louis, MO 63131
800-423-1982
In St. Louis 314-966-6886

Farr Co.
PO Box 92187 (APD)
Airport Station
Los Angeles, CA 90009
800-333-7320
Fax 800-441-0003
and
Farr Co.
500 S. Main Street (APD)
Crystal Lake, IL 60014
800-777-5260
Fax 800-441-0103

Hi-Tech Filter Corp. of America
80 Myrtle St. (APD)
N. Quincy, MA 02171
800-448-3249

In MA 617-328-7756
Fax 617-773-4192

National Allergy Supply, Inc.
4400 Georgia Hwy. 120 (APD)
PO Box 1658 (APD)
Duluth, GA 30136
800-522-1448
In Atlanta 404-623-8077
Fax 404-623-5568

Newtron Products
PO Box 27175 (APD)
3874 Virginia Ave. (APD)
Cincinnati, OH 45227-0175
800-543-9149
In OH 800-544-3753
513-561-7373
Fax 513-561-3673

Permatron Corp.
11400 Melrose St. (APD)
Franklin Park, IL 60131-1325
800-882-8012
708-451-0999

EQUIPMENT REPAIR, LEASING

Entech®
Repairs respiratory equipment in the continental U.S.; mail service
4411 S. 40th St., Ste. 6 (APD)
Phoenix, AZ 85040-2901
800-451-0591
In AZ: 602-437-9081

General Biomedical Service, Inc.
Repairs respiratory equipment in Alabama, Louisiana, Mississippi; sells in the continental U.S. to hospitals, industry, homes; mails with UPS
1000 Riverbend Blvd. #5 (APD)
St. Rose, LA 70087
800-558-9449
504-468-8597

Asthma Resources Directory

Special Services

Med-Electronics

Leases, sells, and repairs parts for air filters, air cleaners, nebuilizers and spirometers in Maryland, Virginia, District of Columbia
9723 Baltimore Ave. #4 (APD)
College Park, MD 20740
301-345-8826
FAX 301-345-5686

Mediq/PRN

Repairs, leases, and sells parts for respiratory equipment for hospital use in the continental U.S.
1 Mediq Plaza (APD)
Pennsauken, NJ 08110
800-257-7477
In NJ: 800-232-6900

New Life Systems, Inc.

Leases, repairs, sells parts, and used respiratory equipment for hospital, industrial, and home use in the continental U.S.
PO Box 8767 (APD)
Coral Springs, FL 33075
Send repairs to:
1870 N. State Rd. 7 (APD)
Margate, FL 33063
305-972-4600
FAX 305-968-1990

Puritan-Bennett Corp.

Repairs and sells parts and respiratory equipment for hospitals, medical care dealers, and homes in the continental U.S. and Canada
Available from:
Puritan-Bennett
900 Springer Dr. (APD)
Lombard, IL 60148-6404
800-255-5444
Regional IL 800-255-6773
Regional GA 404-822-0700
For Home Care 800-248-0890
708-495-5444
Fax 800-755-8075
Fax 708-495-4433

Radiometer America, Inc.

Leases, repairs, and sells parts and used respiratory equipment for hospitals in the continental U.S.
811 Sharon Dr. (APD)
Westlake, OH 44145
800-377-7004
In OH: 216-871-8900

Respiratory Management Services, Inc.

Leases, repairs and sells parts and used respiratory equipment for hospitals, industry, and home in the continental U.S.; parts repaired by UPS
364 Adams St. (APD)
Bedford Hills, NJ 10507
800-431-2460
In NY: 914-666-2990

195

Asthma Resources Directory
Allergy/Asthma Stores

SUPPLIERS OF ALLERGY AND ASTHMA PRODUCTS

A-Plus Equipment & Supply
Products for the air; cotton products; products for the home; respiratory care
Available from:
A-Plus Allergy Equipment & Supply
8325 Regis Way (APD)
Los Angeles, CA 90045-2646
Orders 800-86-ALLER (862-5537)
310-337-7468
Fax 310-337-1971

Absolute Environmental's Allergy Store
Products for the air; products for the home; respiratory care
Available from:
Absolute Environmental's Allergy Store
2615 S. University Dr. (APD)
Davie, FL 33328
Nationwide 800-771-ACHOO (2246)
In FL 800-329-3773
Broward 305-472-3773
Fax 305-474-0133

Aller-Guard®
Products for the air; products for the home
Available from:
Aller-Guard,® Inc.
Southgate Office Park
1645 S.W. 41st St. (APD)
Topeka, KS 66609-1250
800-234-0816
913-267-9333
Fax 913-267-0072

Allergy Aide Centre
Products for the air; products for the home; respiratory care
Available from:
Allergy Aid Centre
1st Floor Pran Central Shop 56
325 Chapel St. (APD)
Prahran, Vic 3181

Australia
03-529-7348
03-529-8459

Allergy Asthma Technology
Products for the air; products for the home; respiratory care
Available from:
Allergy Asthma Technology
4151 N. Kedzie (APD)
PO Box 18398 (APD)
Chicago, IL 60618
800-621-5545
312-465-8020
Fax 312-465-7619

Allergy Clean Environments
Products for the air; products for the home
Available from:
Allergy Clean Environments
501 Station Ave. (APD)
Haddon Heights, NJ 08035
800-882-4110
In NJ 609-546-1101
Fax 609-546-1466
URL:
http:\\WWW.infomall.com\allergy.html

Allergy Control Products, Inc.
Products for the air; products for the home; respiratory care
Available from:
Allergy Control Products, Inc.
96 Danbury Rd. (APD)
PO Box 793 (APD)
Ridgefield, CT 06877
800-422-DUST (3878)
203-438-9580
Fax 203-431-8963

Allergy Relief Products
Products for the air; products for the home; publications
Available from:

Asthma Resources Directory

Allergy/Asthma Stores

Allergy Relief Products
9 Renata Ct. (APD)
Dundas, ON L9H 6X1
Canada
905-628-5324 ?416
Fax 416-628-1734

Allergy Relief Shop, Inc.
Products for the air; products for the home
Available from:
Allergy Relief Shop™ Inc.
3371 Whittle Springs Rd. (APD)
Knoxville, TN 37917
Orders 800-626-2810
Questions 615-522-2795

Allergy Resources
Products for the air; products for the home
Available from:
Allergy Resources
Mail: PO Box 888 (APD)
UPS: 264 Brookridge Ave. (APD)
Palmer Lake, CO 80133
Orders 800-USE-FLAX (873-3529)
Company plans to move; use 800 #

Allergy Shop, Ltd., The
Products for the air; products for the home;
Available from:
Allergy Shop, Ltd.
3420 Cardston Crescent N.W. (APD)
Calgary, AB T2L 0S6
Canada
403-289-9052

Allergy Supply Co., Inc., The
Products for the air; products for the home; respiratory care
Available from:
Allergy Supply Co.
11994 Star Court (APD)
Herndon, VA 22071
800-323-6744
Metropolitan DC 703-391-2011
Fax 703-391-2014
BBS 703-521-0638

Allergy-Asthma Shopper™
Products for the air; products for the home; respiratory care
Available from:
Allergy-Asthma Shopper™
PO Box 239 (APD)
Fate, TX 75132
800-447-1100
Fax 903-883-4513

American Allergy Supply
Products for the air; products for the home; respiratory care
Available from:
PO Box 722022 (APD)
Houston, TX 77272-2022
800-321-1096
713-995-6110

Bermuda Asthma & Allergy Relief Center
Caribbean Asthma & Allergy Relief Center
The Recorder Bldg.
63 Court St. (APD)
Hamilton HM 12
Bermuda
809-292-9258
Fax 809-292-4535

DeVilbiss, Inc.
Products for the air; products for the home; respiratory care
Available from:
Sunrise Medical/DeVilbiss, Inc.
PO Box 635 (APD)
Somerset, PA 15501-0635
800-DeV-1988 (338-1988)
814-443-4881
Fax 800-345-2202
In Canada 705-728-5522

E.L. Foust Company, Inc.
Products for the air; products for the home
Available from:
E.L. Foust Co., Inc.
PO Box 105 (APD)
Elmhurst, IL 60126
800-225-9549

Asthma Resources Directory

Allergy/Asthma Stores

708-834-4952
Fax 708-834-5341

Environtrol®
Products for the air; products for the home
Available from:
Environtrol® Corporation
PO Box 31313 (APD)
St. Louis, MO 63131
800-423-1982
In St. Louis 314-966-6886

Flowright International Products
Products for the air; products for the home
Available from:
Flowright Int'l Products
1495 N.W. Gilman Blvd. #4 (APD)
Issaquah, WA 98027
206-392-8357

N.E.E.D.S.
Products for the air; products for the home; respiratory care
Available from:

N.E.E.D.S.
527 Charles Ave. 12A (APD)
Syrcause, NY 13209
800-634-1380
Fax 800-295-NEED (6333)

National Allergy Supply, Inc.
Products for the air; products for the home; respiratory care
Available from:
National Allergy Supply, Inc.
4400 Georgia Hwy. 120 (APD)
PO Box 1658 (APD)
Duluth, GA 30136
800-522-1448
In Atlanta 404-623-8077
Fax 404-623-5568

Skin & Allergy™ Shop, Inc., The
Available from:
Skin & Allergy Shop,™The
310 E. Broadway (APD)
Louisville, KY 40202
800-366-6483
In KY 502-585-4824
Fax 502-589-3429

Allergy Products Directory
Copyrighted. Reproduction Prohibited by Law. 1259 El Camino #254, Menlo Park, CA 94025

Asthma Resources Directory
Catalogues and Mail Order

CATALOGUES AND MAIL ORDER

AIR FILTERS AND MOLD CONTROL

3M Company
PO Box 33275 (APD)
St. Paul, MN 55133-3275
3M Center Bldg.(APD)
St. Paul, MN 55144-1000
Medical information 800-328-0255
Medical information local 612-736-4930
Customer service 800-423-5197
Outside CA 800-423-5146
In CA 818-341-1300

A-Plus Allergy Equipment & Supply
8325 Regis Way (APD)
Los Angeles, CA 90045-2646
Orders 800-86-ALLER (862-5537)
310-337-7468
Fax 310-337-1971

AAir Purification Systems
7340 Trade St. #C (APD)
San Diego, CA 92121-2457
800-776-6746
619-578-2825
Fax 619-578-3762

Absolute Environmental's Allergy Store
2615 S. University Dr. (APD)
Davie, FL 33328
Nationwide 800-771-ACHOO (2246)
In FL 800-329-3773
Broward 305-472-3773
Fax 305-474-0133

Air Quality Engineering, Inc.
3340 Winpark Dr. (APD)
Minneapolis, MN 55427-2083
800-328-0787
612-544-4426
Fax 612-544-4013

Aireox Research Corp.
11015 Whitford Ave. (APD)
Riverside, CA 92505
909-689-2781

Aller-Guard,® Inc.
Southgate Office Park
1645 S.W. 41st St. (APD)
Topeka, KS 66609-1250
800-234-0816
913-267-9333
Fax 913-267-0072

Allergen™ Air Filter Corp.
5205 Ashbrook (APD)
Houston, TX 77081
800-333-8880
In TX 713-668-2371

Allergy Aid Centre
1st Floor Pran Central Shop 56
325 Chapel St. (APD)
Prahran, Vic 3181
Australia
03-529-7348
03-529-8459

Allergy Asthma Technology
4151 N. Kedzie (APD)
PO Box 18398 (APD)
Chicago, IL 60618
800-621-5545
312-465-8020
Fax 312-465-7619

Allergy Clean Environments
501 Station Ave. (APD)
Haddon Heights, NJ 08035
800-882-4110
In NJ 609-546-1101
Fax 609-546-1466
URL:
http:\\WWW.infomall.com\allergy.html

Allergy Control Products, Inc.
96 Danbury Rd. (APD)
PO Box 793 (APD)

199

Asthma Resources Directory

Catalogues and Mail Order

Ridgefield, CT 06877
800-422-DUST (3878)
203-438-9580
Fax 203-431-8963

Allergy Relief Products
9 Renata Ct. (APD)
Dundas, ON L9H 6X1
Canada
905-628-5324 ?416
Fax 416-628-1734

Allergy Relief Shop™, Inc.
3371 Whittle Springs Rd. (APD)
Knoxville, TN 37917
Orders 800-626-2810
Questions 615-522-2795

Allergy Resources
Mail: PO Box 888 (APD)
UPS: 264 Brookridge Ave. (APD)
Palmer Lake, CO 80133
Orders 800-USE-FLAX (873-3529)
Company plans to move; use 800 #

Allergy Supply Co., Inc., The
11994 Star Court (APD)
Herndon, VA 22071
800-323-6744
Metropolitan DC 703-391-2011
Fax 703-391-2014
BBS 703-521-0638

Allergy-Asthma Shopper™
PO Box 239 (APD)
Fate, TX 75132
800-447-1100
Fax 903-883-4513

Appliance Sales & Service Co.
655 Mission St. (APD)
San Francisco, CA 94105
800-424-6783
In 415 area call 415-362-7195

Brookstone Co.
5 Vose Farm Road (APD)
Peterborough, NH 03458
800-926-7000
Fax 603-924-0093

Cloud 9®
Div. of Mason Engineering Corp.
777 Edgewood Ave. (APD)
Wood Dale, IL 60191
708-595-5000

DeVilbiss
Available from:
Sunrise Medical/DeVilbiss, Inc.
PO Box 635 (APD)
Somerset, PA 15501-0635
800-DeV-1988 (338-1988)
814-443-4881
Fax 800-345-2202
In Canada 705-728-5522

E.L. Foust Co., Inc.
PO Box 105 (APD)
Elmhurst, IL 60126
800-225-9549
708-834-4952
Fax 708-834-5341

Edmund Scientific Co.
101 E. Gloucester Pike (APD)
Barrington, NJ 08007-1380
609-573-6250
Fax 609-573-6295

Honeywell/Enviracaire®
Honeywell Environmental Air Control
100 Jamison Ct. (APD)
Hagerstown, MD 21740-5185
800-332-1110

Environtrol® Corporation
PO Box 31313 (APD)
St. Louis, MO 63131
800-423-1982
In St. Louis 314-966-6886

Flowright Int'l Products
1495 N.W. Gilman Blvd. #4 (APD)
Issaquah, WA 98027
206-392-8357

Gempler's
211 Blue Mounds Rd. (APD)
PO Box 270 (APD)
Mt. Horeb, WI 53572

Asthma Resources Directory
Catalogues and Mail Order

800-382-8473
Fax 800-551-1128

Hammacher Schlemmer
Heaters, mold control, bedding
Available from:
Hammacher Schlemmer
147 E. 57th St. (APD)
New York, NY 10022
800-543-3366
212-421-9000

Herrington
3 Symmes Dr. (APD)
Londonderry, NH 03053
800-622-5221
In NH 603-437-4939
603-437-4638

Hi-Tech Filter Corp. of America
80 Myrtle St. (APD)
N. Quincy, MA 02171
800-448-3249
In MA 617-328-7756
Fax 617-773-4192

Holmes Products Corp.
233 Fortune Blvd. (APD)
Milford, MA 01757
508-634-8050
Fax 508-634-1211

King-Aire®
1121 S.R. 32 E. (APD)
Noblesville, IN 46060
Mail to PO Box 398 (APD)
Noblesville, IN 46060-0398
800-999-KING (5464)
317-776-1600

N.E.E.D.S.
527 Charles Ave. 12A (APD)
Syracuse, NY 13209
800-634-1380
Fax 800-295-NEED (6333)

National Allergy Supply, Inc.
4400 Georgia Hwy. 120 (APD)
PO Box 1658 (APD)
Duluth, GA 30136

800-522-1448
In Atlanta 404-623-8077
Fax 404-623-5568

Newtron Products
PO Box 27175 (APD)
3874 Virginia Ave. (APD)
Cincinnati, OH 45227-0175
800-543-9149
In OH 800-544-3753
513-561-7373
Fax 513-561-3673

Research Products, Corp.
1015 E. Washington Ave. (APD)
PO Box 1467 (APD)
Madison, WI 53701-1467
800-545-2219
608-257-8801
Fax 608-257-4357

Skin & Allergy Shop,™ The
310 E. Broadway (APD)
Louisville, KY 40202
800-366-6483
In KY 502-585-4824
Fax 502-589-3429

Sporty's® Preferred Living
Clermont County Airport (APD)
Batavia, OH 45103-9747
800-543-8633
Fax 513-732-6560

Tectronic Products Co., Inc.
PO Box 157 (APD)
6500 Badgley Rd. (APD)
E. Syracuse, NY 13057-0157
800-227-1375
315-463-0240
Fax 315-437-7290

HELP US TO HELP YOU
When writing to the companies
and organizations listed here, be sure
to use the initials (APD) as part of the
address and tell them you saw them
listed in *Allergy Products Directory.*

Asthma Resources Directory

Catalogues and Mail Order

COTTON CLOTHING AND HOUSEHOLD SUPPLIES

A-Plus Allergy Equipment & Supply
8325 Regis Way (APD)
Los Angeles, CA 90045-2646
Orders 800-86-ALLER (862-5537)
310-337-7468
Fax 310-337-1971

Allergy Relief Shop™, Inc.
3371 Whittle Springs Rd. (APD)
Knoxville, TN 37917
Orders 800-626-2810
Questions 615-522-2795

Allergy Resources
Mail: PO Box 888 (APD)
UPS: 264 Brookridge Ave. (APD)
Palmer Lake, CO 80133
Orders 800-USE-FLAX (873-3529)
Company plans to move; use 800 #

Allergy-Asthma Shopper™
PO Box 239 (APD)
Fate, TX 75132
800-447-1100
Fax 903-883-4513

Australian Conservation Foundation
340 Gore St. (APD)
Fitzroy Vic 3065
Australia
(03)-416-1166
008-332-510

Childcraft, Inc.
PO Box 29149 (APD)
Mission, KS 66201
800-631-5657
Fax 913-752-1095

Clothcrafters, Inc.
PO Box 176 (APD)
Elkhart Lake, WI 53020
414-876-2112
Fax 800-876-2009

Comfortably Yours
2515 E. 43rd St. (APD)
Chattanooga, TN 37422
201-368-0400

Cotton On Clothing Co., Ltd., The
Monmouth Place (APD)
Bath BA1 2NP
England
44-022-546-1155
Fax-44-022-546-1464

Domestications
PO Box 40 (APD)
Hanover, PA 17333-0040
800-746-2555

Dona Designs
1611 Bent Tree St. (APD)
Seagoville, TX 75159
214-287-7834
Don & Dona Shrier

French Creek
RD #1 (APD)
Elverson, PA 19520-0110
215-286-5700

Janice Corp.
198 US Hwy. 46 (APD)
Budd Lake, NJ 07828-3001
800-JANICES (526-4237)
Fax 201-691-5459

L.L. Bean, Inc.
Freeport, ME 04033
800-221-4221

Lands' End & Coming Home
1 Lands' End Ln. (APD
Dodgeville, WI 53595
800-345-3696
TDD 800-541-3459

N.E.E.D.
527 Charles Ave 12A (APD)
Syracuase, NY 13209
800-634-1380
Fax 800-295-NEED (6333)

PlayClothes, Inc.

Asthma Resources Directory
Catalogues and Mail Order

PO Box 29137 (APD)
Overland Park, KS 66201-9137
800-362-PLAY (7529)
Fax 913-752-1095

Primary Layer, The
PO Box 6697 (APD)
Portland, OR 97228
800-282-8206

S&H® Uniform Corp.
200 Wiliam St. (APD)
Port Chester, NY 10573
914-937-6800
Fax 914-937-00741

HOUSEHOLD AND PERSONAL AIDS

A-Plus Allergy Equipment & Supply
8325 Regis Way (APD)
Los Angeles, CA 90045-2646
Orders 800-86-ALLER (862-5537)
310-337-7468
Fax 310-337-1971

Absolute Environmental's Allergy Store
2615 S. University Dr. (APD)
Davie, FL 33328
Nationwide 800-771-ACHOO (2246)
In FL 800-329-3773
Broward 305-472-3773
Fax 305-474-0133

Aller-Guard,® Inc.
Southgate Office Park
1645 S.W. 41st St. (APD)
Topeka, KS 66609-1250
800-234-0816
913-267-9333
Fax 913-267-0072

Allergy Aid Centre
1st Floor Pran Central Shop 56
325 Chapel St. (APD)
Prahran, Vic 3181
Australia

03-529-7348
03-529-8459

Allergy Clean Environments
501 Station Ave. (APD)
Haddon Heights, NJ 08035
800-882-4110
In NJ 609-546-1101
Fax 609-546-1466
URL:
http:\\WWW.infomall.com\allergy.html

Allergy Control Products, Inc.
96 Danbury Rd. (APD)
PO Box 793 (APD)
Ridgefield, CT 06877
800-422-DUST (3878)
203-438-9580
Fax 203-431-8963

Allergy Relief Distributors
Div. of E.C.Environmental Control, Inc.
177 Telegraph Rd. #365 (APD)
Bellingham, WA 98226
206-734-1646
Fax 206-734-3696
Canadian office in Vancouver, BC

Allergy Relief Products
9 Renata Ct. (APD)
Dundas, ON L9H 6X1
Canada
905-628-5324 ?416
Fax 416-628-1734

Allergy Relief Shop™, Inc.
3371 Whittle Springs Rd. (APD)
Knoxville, TN 37917
Orders 800-626-2810
Questions 615-522-2795

Allergy Resources
Mail: PO Box 888 (APD)
UPS: 264 Brookridge Ave. (APD)
Palmer Lake, CO 80133
Orders 800-USE-FLAX (873-3529)
Company plans to move; use 800 #

Asthma Resources Directory

Catalogues and Mail Order

Allergy Supply Co.
11994 Star Court (APD)
Herndon, VA 22071
800-323-6744
Metropolitan DC 703-391-2011
Fax 703-391-2014
BBS 703-521-0638

Allergy-Asthma Shopper™
PO Box 239 (APD)
Fate, TX 75132
800-447-1100
Fax 903-883-4513

Apex™ Medical Corp.
800 S. Van Eps Ave. (APD)
Sioux Falls, SD 57104
PO Box 1235 (APD)
Sioux Falls, SD 57101
800-328-2935
In SD 605-332-6689
Fax 605-332-6818

Ar-Ex Ltd.
156 N. Jefferson St. #205 (APD)
Chicago, IL 60661
312-879-0017
Fax 312-879-0019

Aussie Wool Quilts & Pillows
RMB 2276 (APD)
Bullswamp Rd.
Warragul Sth. 3820
Australia
056-26-1242

Brookstone Co.
5 Vose Farm Road (APD)
Peterborough, NH 03458
800-926-7000
Fax 603-924-0093

Conney Safety Products
3203 Latham Dr. (APD)
PO Box 44190 (APD)
Madison, WI 53744-4190
800-356-9100
Fax 800-845-9095

Consolidated Plastics Co., Inc.
8181 Darrow Rd. (APD)
Twinsburg, OH 44087
800-362-1000
216-425-3900
Fax 216-425-3333

DeVilbiss
Available from:
Sunrise Medical/DeVilbiss, Inc.
PO Box 635 (APD)
Somerset, PA 15501-0635
800-DeV-1988 (338-1988)
814-443-4881
Fax 800-345-2202
In Canada 705-728-5522

Direct Safety Co.
7815 S. 46th St. (APD)
Phoenix, AZ 85044-5399
PO Box 50050 (APD)
Phoenix, AZ 85076-0050
800-528-7405
In AZ 602-968-7009
Fax 800-366-9662

Discount Safety
Available from:
Interex Safety & Industrial Supplies
176 Newington Rd. (APD)
W. Hartford, CT 06110
800-225-5910
Fax 800-334-2594

Dona Designs
1611 Bent Tree St. (APD)
Seagoville, TX 75159
214-287-7834
Don & Dona Shrier

E.L. Foust Co., Inc.
PO Box 105 (APD)
Elmhurst, IL 60126
800-225-9549
708-834-4952
Fax 708-834-5341

Environtrol® Corporation
PO Box 31313 (APD)
St. Louis, MO 63131

Asthma Resources Directory
Catalogues and Mail Order

800-423-1982
In St. Louis 314-966-6886

Flowright Int'l Products
1495 N.W. Gilman Blvd. #4 (APD)
Issaquah, WA 98027
206-392-8357

Gempler's
211 Blue Mounds Rd. (APD)
PO Box 270 (APD)
Mt. Horeb, WI 53572
800-382-8473
Fax 800-551-1128

Hammacher Schlemmer
147 E. 57th St. (APD)
New York, NY 10022
800-543-3366
212-421-9000

Industrial Safety Co.
1390 Neubrecht Rd. (APD)
Lima, OH 45801-3196
Orders 800-537-9721
Customer Service 419-227-6030
Fax 419-228-5034

Janice Corp.
198 US Hwy. 46 (APD)
Budd Lake, NJ 07828-3001
800-JANICES (526-4237)
Fax 201-691-5459

N.E.E.D.S.
527 Charles Ave. 12A (APD)
Syracuse, NY 13209
800-634-1380
Fax 800-295-NEED (6333)

National Allergy Supply, Inc.
4400 Georgia Hwy. 120 (APD)
PO Box 1658 (APD)
Duluth, GA 30136
800-522-1448
In Atlanta 404-623-8077
Fax 404-623-5568

Rx Systems, Inc.
#20 Point West Blvd. (APD)

St. Charles, MO 63301
800-922-9142
Fax 314-925-0041

Skin & Allergy Shop™, The
310 E. Broadway (APD)
Louisville, KY 40202
800-366-6483
In KY 502-585-4824
Fax 502-589-3429

Solutions®
PO Box 6878 (APD)
Portland, OR 97228
800-342-9988
Fax 503-643-1973

Sun Precautions, Inc.
2815 Wetmore Ave. (APD)
Everett, WA 98201
800-882-7860
206-303-8585
Fax 206-303-0836

Touch of Class
1905 N. Van Buren St. (APD)
Huntingburg, IN 47542-9595
800-457-7456
Fax 812-683-5921

West Coast Shoe Co.
52828 N.W. Shoe Factory Ln. (APD)
PO Box 607 (APD)
Scappoose, OR 97056-0607
800-326-2711
503-543-7114
Fax 503-543-7110

RESPIRATORY TOOLS

Absolute Environmental's Allergy Store
2615 S. University Dr. (APD)
Davie, FL 33328
Nationwide 800-771-ACHOO (2246)
In FL 800-329-3773
Broward 305-472-3773
Fax 305-474-0133

Asthma Resources Directory

Catalogues and Mail Order

Aller-Guard,® Inc.
Southgate Office Park
1645 S.W. 41st St. (APD)
Topeka, KS 66609-1250
800-234-0816
913-267-9333
Fax 913-267-0072

Allergy Aid Centre
1st Floor Pran Central Shop 56
325 Chapel St. (APD)
Prahran, Vic 3181
Australia
03-529-7348
03-529-8459

Allergy Control Products, Inc.
96 Danbury Rd. (APD)
PO Box 793 (APD)
Ridgefield, CT 06877
800-422-DUST (3878)
203-438-9580
Fax 203-431-8963

Allergy Supply Co.
11994 Star Court (APD)
Herndon, VA 22071
800-323-6744
Metropolitan DC 703-391-2011
Fax 703-391-2014
BBS 703-521-0638

Allergy-Asthma Shopper™
PO Box 239 (APD)
Fate, TX 75132
800-447-1100
Fax 903-883-4513

Conney Safety Products
3203 Latham Dr. (APD)
PO Box 44190 (APD)
Madison, WI 53744-4190
800-356-9100
Fax 800-845-9095

Consolidated Plastics Co., Inc.
8181 Darrow Rd. (APD)
Twinsburg, OH 44087
800-362-1000
216-425-3900

Fax 216-425-3333

DeVilbiss
Available from:
Sunrise Medical/DeVilbiss, Inc.
PO Box 635 (APD)
Somerset, PA 15501-0635
800-DeV-1988 (338-1988)
814-443-4881
Fax 800-345-2202
In Canada 705-728-5522

Direct Safety Co.
7815 S. 46th St. (APD)
Phoenix, AZ 85044-5399
PO Box 50050 (APD)
Phoenix, AZ 85076-0050
800-528-7405
In AZ 602-968-7009
Fax 800-366-9662

N.E.E.D.S.
527 Charles Ave. 12A (APD)
Syracuse, NY 13209
800-634-1380
Fax 800-295-NEED (6333)

National Allergy Supply, Inc.
4400 Georgia Hwy. 120 (APD)
PO Box 1658 (APD)
Duluth, GA 30136
800-522-1448
In Atlanta 404-623-8077
Fax 404-623-5568

Skin & Allergy Shop,™ The
310 E. Broadway (APD)
Louisville, KY 40202
800-366-6483
In KY 502-585-4824
Fax 502-589-3429

WORK ENVIRONMENTS

Airgard, Inc.
12601 Pleasant Grove #10 (APD)
Syracuse, IN 46567
219-457-5237

Asthma Resources Directory
Catalogues and Mail Order

Allerderm Laboratories, Inc.
PO Box 2070 (APD)
Petaluma, CA 94953-2070
800-365-6868
707-765-6868
Fax 800-926-4568

Allied Glove & Safety Products Corp.
4711 W. Armitage Ave. (APD)
Chicago, IL 60639
800-621-3861
312-804-1800
Fax 312-804-1810

Conney Safety Products
3203 Latham Dr. (APD)
PO Box 44190 (APD)
Madison, WI 53744-4190
800-356-9100
Fax 800-845-9095

Gempler's
211 Blue Mounds Rd. (APD)
PO Box 270 (APD)
Mt. Horeb, WI 53572
800-382-8473
Fax 800-551-1128

Industrial Safety Co.
1390 Neubrecht Rd. (APD)
Lima, OH 45801-3196
Orders 800-537-9721
Customer Service 419-227-6030
Fax 419-228-5034

Interex Safety & Industrial Supplies
176 Newington Rd. (APD)
W. Hartford, CT 06110

800-225-5910
Fax 800-334-2594

Masuen™ Co.
490 Fillmore Ave. (A{D)
Tonawanda, NY 14150
800-831-0894
In IL 312-956-1255
Fax 800-222-1934

Medical Equipment Designs, Inc.
23461 Ridge Route Dr. #F (APD)
Laguna Hills, CA 92653
800-323-1674
714-859-7779

Pioneer Industrial Products
512 E. Tiffin St. (APD)
Willard, OH 44890
800-537-2897
In OH 419-933-2211
Fax 419-933-2710
Telex 210-498-2691

RH Hinchliffe & Sons, Ltd.
58 Bridge St. (APD)
Pershore
Worcestershire WR10 3AX
England

St. George Co., Ltd.
20 Consolidated Dr. (APD)
PO Box 430 (APD)
Paris, ON N3L 3T5
Canada
519-442-2046
Fax 519-442-7191
U.S. 800-461-4299

Allergy Products Directory

Copyrighted. Reproduction Prohibited by Law. 1259 El Camino #254,Menlo Park, CA 94025

Asthma Resources Directory

Environmental Smoke

TOBACCO SMOKE IN THE ENVIRONMENT

United States Environmental Protection Agency
Office of Air and Radiation

Environmental tobacco smoke is a widespread indoor air pollutant. It comes from secondhand smoke exhaled by smokers and the sidestream smoke from the burning ends of cigarettes, cigars, and pipes. It is a mixture of irritating gases and carcinogenic tar particles.

Symptoms from secondhand smoke are coughing, phlegm, reduced lung function, and itching and watering of the eyes. An estimated 3,000 nonsmoking Americans die annually from lung cancer caused by secondhand smoke.

1986 SURGEON GENERAL'S REPORT

In 1985, the US Public Health Service under the Surgeon General, the National Research Council, and the Interagency Task Force and Environmental Cancer, Heart, and Lung Disease convened to consider the public health implications of passive smoking.

In the 1986 Surgeon General's report participants arrived at the following consensus:

Passive smoking (breathing in environmental tobacco smoke) significantly increases the risk of lung cancer in adults.

Passive smoking (breathing in environmental tobacco smoke) significantly increases the risk of lung cancer in adults.

Passive smoking increases respiratory illness in children.

From the Surgeon General: "A substantial number of the lung cancer deaths that occur among nonsmokers can be attributed to involuntary smoking."

•   Physical separation of smokers and nonsmokers even in different rooms of the same house may reduce but not eliminate nonsmoker's exposure to environmental tobacco smoke.

•   There was further agreement that passive smoking substantially increases respiratory illness in children.

Allergy Products Directory
Copyrighted. Reproduction Prohibited by Law. 1259 El Camino #254, Menlo Park, CA 94025

Asthma Resources Directory
Environmental Smoke

EPA, SURGEON GENERAL 1986 CONCLUSIONS

In 1986, the Surgeon General's Report concluded that:

1. Adults should not expose children to environmental smoke.

2. Employers should restrict smoking to separately ventilated areas or ban smoking from buildings.

EPA 1991 CONCLUSIONS

In 1991, the Science Advisory Board reported to the Environmental Protection Agency (EPA) that secondhand tobacco smoke should be declared a Class A carcinogen.

In 1992, the EPA and its Science Advisory Board, after extensive study, published the following conclusions:

✔ Widespread exposure to environmental tobacco smoke in the U.S. is a serious public health risk.

✔ Environmental tobacco smoke is a human lung carcinogen, responsible for approximately 3,000 lung cancer deaths annually in non-smokers.

✔ Environmental tobacco smoke impairs the respiratory health of hundreds of thousands of children. When parents smoke with children present, the children are at increased risk of lower respiratory tract infections and are more likely to have symptoms of respiratory irritation like cough, excess phlegm, and wheezing.

EPA
401 M St., SW, Washington, DC 20460
202-260-2090
Telnet epaibm.rtpnc.epa.gov

ORGANIZATIONS LOOK AT SECONDHAND SMOKE

Recently, the Harvard School of Public Health looked at lung tissue and the history of 400 individuals who had been killed or died in accidents. Forty-one of them were women. Seventeen of the women had been married to husbands who smoked; thirteen were married to nonsmokers and 11 were unidentified.

There were more abnormalities in the lungs of the wives of the smokers than in the wives of the nonsmokers.

The significance here is that there could be no bias in collecting the data. These individuals were of Greek nationality and autopsies are mandatory in cases of death from external causes.

Asthma Resources Directory

Environmental Smoke

Health organizations like the National Academy of Sciences and the American Medical Association note that secondhand smoke is a serious factor in heart attack death.

Journal of the American Medical Association has also written that women who lived with smokers had a 30% increased risk of lung cancer with exposure to a moderate amount of secondhand smoke. If these women lived with a heavy smoker, the risk increased to 80%. Even at work, risk was 39% increased.

STUDIES LOOK AT CHILDREN'S EXPOSURE TO SECONDHAND SMOKE

✔ A study of infants with bronchiolitis was initiated to look for expectancy of long-term pulmonary problems. When the infants were seven years old, they were given skin tests and pulmonary testing. Several of these children had mild pulmonary dysfunction significantly correlated with exposure to others smoking. (*Journal of Allergy & Clinical Immunology* 1994. vol 89 no. 1)

✔ Children exposed to secondhand smoke are more likely to spend more time in emergency rooms, more likely to develop ear infections and lower respiratory tract infections, asthma, bronchitis, and pneumonia according to the American Academy of Otolaryngology-Head and Neck Surgery.

✔ Another study looked at children with allergic dermatitis (eczema) and discovered that these children were more likely to develop asthma if their mothers smoked. In general, children with a smoking parent are more likely to develop asthma, but this was the first study to show that children who have allergic dermatitis are more likely to develop asthma if the mother smoked. (*Journal of Allergy & Clinical Immunology* 1991 vol 86 no. 5)

Children exposed to secondhand smoke are more likely to spend more time in emergency rooms.
They are more likely to develop asthma, bronchitis, and pneumonia.

—American Academy of Otolaryngology-Head and Neck Surgery

✔ Children with asthma are particularly at risk and children of smokers have significantly higher rates of hospitalization for bronchitis and other respiratory problems, especially up to the age of two. Further, children of women who smoked during pregnancy were more likely to develop asthma than children of women who did not smoke. (*Pediatrics.* 4/90)

✔ Another study has examined children with asthma. Researchers at Mt. Sinai Medical Center in New York looked at the histories of over 200 children; half of them had asthma, half did not. Those with asthma were 50 percent more likely to have mothers who smoked.

The investigators wanted to be sure that their results were accurate and so they gave the children urine tests, looking for a byproduct of nicotine. Children with asthma had levels 69 percent higher than children without asthma.

The researchers conclusion was that children were twice as likely to develop asthma if they had been exposed to secondhand smoke. (*American Review of Respiratory Disease.* 3/92)

Children were twice as likely to develop asthma if they had been exposed to secondhand smoke.

✔ The 1992 report by the Environmental Protection Agency concluded that up to one million asthma attacks and up to 300,000 cases of bronchitis and pneumonia in infants, children, and adolescents are caused each year by exposure to secondhand smoke. The agency declared secondhand smoke to be a Class A Carcinogen.

EPA has delcared secondhand smoke to be a Class A Carcinogen.

IMPACT ON CHILDREN

Passive smoking induces serious respiratory symptoms in children. Wheezing, coughing and sputum production among children of smoking parents increase by 20 percent to 80 percent depending upon the symptom and the number of smokers in the household.

Perhaps 300,000 infections a year in children under eighteen months of age can be attributed to exposure to secondhand smoke. These children are more likely to be hospitalized — between 7,500 and 15,000 according to the Centers for Disease Control and Prevention.

EPA estimates that between 200,000 and 1,000,000 asthmatic children have their condition made worse by exposure to secondhand smoke each each. EPA estimates that passive smoking causes between 150,000 and 300,000 lower respiratory tract infections in infants and children

Asthma Resources Directory

Environmental Smoke

under 18 months of age, resulting in between 7,500 and 15,000 hospitalizations each year.

Exposure to environmental tobacco smoke is a risk factor
for children to develop asthma
even though they have had no previous symptoms.

In 1992, after extensive study, the EPA and its Science Advisory Board published the following conclusions:

✔ Children with asthma are at particular risk. EPA estimates that exposure to secondhand smoke increases the number and severity of symptoms in children with asthma.

✔ Environmental tobacco smoke raises the risk of lower respiratory tract infections like bronchitis and pneumonia.

✔ In children, exposure to environmental tobacco smoke increases problems with fluid in the middle ear.

✔ In children, exposure to environmental tobacco smoke increases the severity of asthma symptoms and their frequency. EPA estimates 200,000 to 1,000,000 asthmatic children are worse because of this exposure.

✔ Exposure to environmental tobacco smoke is a risk factor for children to develop asthma even though they have had no previous symptoms.

CURRENT PROBLEMS

Barriers or spatial separation of smokers from non-smokers do not eliminate non-smokers' exposure to tobacco smoke. Separating them into different rooms with the same ventilation system may reduce exposure, but does not eliminate it, especially in public buildings where air systems recirculate much of the contaminated indoor air.

Airplanes using barriers to separate smokers still have pollutants circulating through common air space and air systems which recirculate air.

Further, the non-smoking ban does not cover the cockpit and the air there does circulate throughout the plane.

Asthma Resources Directory

Environmental Smoke

WHAT CAN YOU DO AT HOME?

Smoking should not be allowed in your home or car. Be sure that friends, relatives, baby sitters, repair and maintenance personnel do not smoke in your home. Remember that your draperies, upholstery, and carpeting catch particles and the odor remains in your home long after the cigarette is extinguished.

If you smoke, Stop!

Protect your child from exposure to environmental smoke.

Opening windows and using exhaust fans reduces but does not eliminate exposure.

Do not allow smoking in your home and protect your child from exposure outside your home. This includes day care centers, schools, baby sitters, and extra-curricular activities.

Protect yourself from exposure to environmental smoke. Remember that opening windows and using exhaust fans reduces but does not eliminate exposure. Do not allow smoking in your home and avoid such exposure outside your home.

If you smoke. **Stop.**

WHAT CAN YOU DO WHEN EATING OUT?

IN RESTAURANTS

Ask if the restaurant has a non-smoking section. Some areas of the country have stricter restaurant smoking rules than others, and some areas have no regulations at all. Regulations may change between county and incorporated areas. So always ask before you are seated.

Remember that barriers or spatial separation of smokers from non-smokers does not eliminate non-smokers' exposure to tobacco smoke.

Remember that barriers or spatial separation of smokers from non-smokers does not eliminate non-smokers' exposure to tobacco smoke.

Separating separating smokers and non-smokers into different rooms with the same ventilation system may reduce exposure, but does not eliminate it, especially where air systems recirculate much of the contaminated indoor air.

213

Asthma Resources Directory

Environmental Smoke

If the restaurant has a non-smoking area, ask yourself the following questions:

Is it a small area?

Is it surrounded by the smoking area?

Is it protected with physical barriers and is it protected by an appropriate circulation system?

Where is the smoking area? (You don't want to be the first non-smoking table next to the smoking section.)

Is smoke drifting in the air?

Is the atmosphere of the restaurant smoky and hazy?

Other alternatives are to fix simple meals in your room, try room service, or order in. Also, try eating earlier or later to avoid the crowds and the consequent larger number of smokers. A picnic can be a pleasant alternative.

There are alternatives to eating in smoke-filled restaurants.

What are the alternatives if local ordinances do not protect you from smoke in restaurants?

—You can picnic

—You can shop and fix simple meals in your room

—You can try room service

—You can order in

—You can eat earlier or later than the usual mealtimes to avoid the crowds and the consequent larger number of smokers

---

IN FAST FOOD RESTAURANTS

Fast food restaurants generally have small one-room dining areas and one or two smokers are sufficient to fill the area with smoke. Sitting in the non-smoking area, if there is one, is of little help. The only non-smoking area that is truly protected from all the smoke is the seat in your car.

Asthma Resources Directory

Environmental Smoke

ASH Smoking and Health Review reports that the National Council of Chain Restaurants has endorsed the idea of smoking bans in all public places, thanks to the efforts of Action on Smoking and Health.

Some fast food chains have declared restaurants that they own to be non-smoking. However, some restaurants are not company owned, they are franchises, so always check before entering.

Congratulations to McDonald's, Arby's, Dairy Queen, and Check E. Cheese, and others. They do not allow smoking in the restaurants that they own. (Independently owned franchises set their own policies.)

IN CHAIN RESTAURANTS

ASH Smoking and Health Review reports that the National Council of Chain Restaurants has endorsed the idea of smoking bans in all public places, thanks to the efforts of Action on Smoking and Health.

WHAT CAN YOU DO WHEN TRAVELING?

IN HOTEL ROOMS

Call for advance reservations and ask for non-smoker's rooms. There are a limited number of them available in various hotels, but they are not necessarily guaranteed. You'll find the policies of a number of hotel chains listed in this handbook.

Remember that non-smoking room policies may be in place, but cannot necessarily be enforced.

Remember that non-smoking room policies may be in place, but cannot necessarily be enforced. Visitors to the room may smoke and the occupant may smoke. In general, such rooms have been cleaned thoroughly and do not have ashtrays in them and should not have the lingering odor of smoke in draperies, carpets, or bedding.

The rise of non-smoking rooms has lead to a major problem. The smoking rooms are used more intensively by smokers and may tend to have a very heavy odor, which is difficult to eradiate. When rooms were used randomly by smokers and non-smokers, one room generally did not house a concentration of smokers. Be very aware of taking a smoking room when a non-smoking room is not available.

215

Asthma Resources Directory

Environmental Smoke

ON BUS AND AMTRAK

Nowadays, most tour companies are aware of the problem of passengers smoking in enclosed, confined areas and ban smoking on their buses. You can continue to avoid smokers by sitting at smaller tables and telling other passengers you are a non-smoker when they wish to sit at your table.

Before embarking on bus or train tour,
ask the tour operator about the bus smoking policy.

Ask for the policy in writing before signing up.

Before embarking on such a tour, ask the tour operator about the bus smoking policy. Ask for the policy in writing before signing up.

For longer train trips, Amtrak's schedule indicates which trains are smoke-free. This policy should be enforced but if there is smoking and you are unable to obtain satisfaction during the trip, write to

Amtrak Customer Relations
60 Massachusetts Ave., NE, (APD)
Washington, DC 20002
202-906-3000
Fax 202-906-3865

If an Amtrak schedules a train as smoke-free and it isn't, you should also write to Amtrak Customer Relations.

CAR TRAVEL

When traveling by car, try to find non-smoking rooms and eat in non-smoking areas of restaurants. Some areas of the country have more stringent restaurant smoking rules than others.

If you are traveling in an area where non-smoking areas are small, are surrounded by smoking areas, or are not protected with physical barriers, you may find it better to follow our restaurant rules and picnic more often, fix simple meals in your room, try room service, or order in. Also, try eating earlier or later to avoid the crowds and the consequent larger number of smokers.

AIRPORTS

In domestic airport waiting areas, non-smoking areas are being better marked. Unfortunately, airline personnel

216

Asthma Resources Directory

Environmental Smoke

do not always enforce violations. When we've asked them to enforce, they say that the restriction is an airport restriction and not the responsibility of the airline. If you complain, you may be told to call the police yourself in order to enforce the restriction.

Some airports now have smoking rooms. Avoid sitting in their vicinity, since the smoke levels in those rooms are so high, the smell is very strong outside the rooms for a distance of several feet.

You'll find many airports are non-smoking at the gate areas and more airport restaurants are smoke-free.

Waiting areas in some foreign airports are still a problem. Some countries have no non-smoking separation at all and others do not enforce separation nor will they take action on a smoking violation if you complain. You may find a mask of some help.

AIRLINES

Information on airline smoking policies changes almost daily as airlines inaugurate non-smoking test flights to various locations. It is likely that this segment of the market will be in flux for some time to come, although the trend at this time is towards increasing the number of non-smoking flights since ridership is not declining on these flights. In response, airlines are experimenting with more scheduled smoke-free flights.

Foreign airlines are also experimenting with nono-smoking flights in various markets, both domestic and international. For accurate, up-to-date information, you should talk to the airline before booking.

There is no smoking on nonstop flights between the U.S., Canada, Australia, and New Zealand.

SMOKE-FREE AIRLINES:

✔ Delta Airlines

✔ Air Canada has had non-smoking flights since 1991 in foreign flights, including flights to Asia

✔ Air New Zealand is non-smoking in most of its international flights

✔ Cathay Pacific Airways is planning to be all non-smoking before the end of 1995

✔ Singapore Airlines bans smoking on most of its flights, except those to Japan

217

Asthma Resources Directory

Environmental Smoke

✔ American, British Airways, Continental, KLM royal Dutch Airlines, Northwest, TWA, United, and USAir may seek to mutually ban smoking on Atlalntic flights, but first must receive immunity from an antitrust violation.

AIRPLANES

In airplanes, try to avoid being seated near the galley where flight attendants may be smoking, even if you are in non-smoking. Apparently, this is against the policy of some airlines, yet smoking by personnel does occur from time to time in non-smoking sections.

When traveling by airplane, domestic flights are non-smoking. Overseas flights allow smoking and so do many foreign airlines. *Delta Airlines is the first American airline to be completely smoke-free in both its foreign and domestic flights.*

Barriers that separate smokers from non-smokers do not eliminate non-smokers' exposure to tobacco smoke.

For flights that allow smoking, do your best to arrange for a seat in a non-smoking area, in the middle of the section to lessen your chances of exposure to drifting smoke. First class and business class sections are small and it is difficult to avoid smoke exposure there.

> Being in a non-smoking area doesn't protect you from exposure to smoke from other passenger's (and crew's) cigarettes. A National Cancer Institute study (noted in Journal of the American Medical Assn.) indicated that exposure to nicotine in some areas of the plane, even though they were non-smoking areas, was the same as if the passenger was sitting in a smoking section.

Barriers or spatial separation of smokers from non-smokers does not eliminate non-smokers' exposure to tobacco smoke. Airplanes using barriers to separate smokers still have pollutants circulating through common air space and through air systems which recirculate air.

Remember that there are no minimum ventilation standards for cabins. FAA only indicates that cabins are to be "ventilated."

Remember that there are no minimum ventilation standards for airplane cabins.

FAA only indicates that cabins are to be "ventilated."

Asthma Resources Directory

Environmental Smoke

Although an airplane may have 30 air changes per hour, it is the amount of fresh air you receive while on an airplane is important. If the airplane has narrow, tightly, placed seats *and* a narrow body, the volume of air per person may be low. Depending upon the amount of air that is recirculated, the volume of fresh air you receive can be low.

An important difference in exposure to passengers is whether the plane uses 100% fresh air circulation or whether the plane uses recircualted air along with fresh air and what the percentages of each are.

Unfortunately, newer aircraft use more recirculated air – as high as 50% in some planes. It is more fuel efficient.

Be sure to ask the flight attendant to have the ventilation system turned on all the way. Unfortunately, we have observed such a request being politely made and answered very rudely without opportunity for explanation. We later found out the person making the request had asthma and was feeling very uncomfortable.

If something like this should happen to you. . .

HOW TO COMPLAIN

Don't let these events pass without notice. Complain to the:

✔ Airline involved

✔ Association of Flight Attendants
1625 Massachusetts Ave. NW 3rd Flr.
Washington, DC 20036
800-424-2401
202-328-5400
Fax 202-328-5424

✔ Federal Aviation Administration, Flight Standards
800 Independence Ave. SW Rm. 302
Washington, DC 20591-0001
800-32-7873
202-267-3484
Fax 202-267-3505

✔ Your congressional representatives

Complain with restraint. You want your voice to be heard.

USE THE FOLLOWING AS A GUIDE

1. State the facts plainly: the date, the airline, the flight number, the name of the flight attendant

Asthma Resources Directory

Environmental Smoke

2. Describe the situation, what your request was and why you made it, how your request was handled and by whom.

3. Write down the reply or the results at the time of the incident. At the bottom of your letter, list the other agencies or persons that your letter is also going to.

4. If you can, try to select the plane you fly on based on fresh air circulation according to the manufacturer. Sometimes an airline will fly different equipment to the same destination, only at different flight times.

Action on Smoking and Health has an "Airline Complaint Kit" which may be of help to you. Call 202-659-4310.

IN THE FUTURE

The International Civil Aviation Organization (ICAO), an agency of the U.N., voted to urge its more than 150 members to ban smoking on all airline flights by 1996. The resolution noted that members should begin restricting smoking progressively on all international passenger flights as soon as possible.

Currently, it is unknown how this resolution will be accepted and by which airlines and to what extent.

CRUISE TRAVEL

Cruise lines have begun to experiment with smoking policies. These policies are currently in a state of flux and for accurate, up-to-date information, you should talk to the cruise line before booking.

There are two major problems with cruise line smoking policies.

✔ Their 800 number representatives do not give consistent information. We have called several companies three and sometimes five times and have received different answers about smoking policy.

Sometimes representatives tell us that they simply do not have any non-smoking areas, except scattered throughout the dining room. Supervisors then tell us that there *are* non-smoking areas.

We have even received written confirmation of smoking policies and then called the 800 number only to be told something other than what the letter indicated.

Allergy Products Directory

Copyrighted. Reproduction Prohibited by Law. 1259 El Camino #254,Menlo Park, CA 94025

Asthma Resources Directory

Environmental Smoke

✔ Policy is one thing, but enforcement and implementation once on board is another. Frequently, ship personnel do not enforce non-smoking areas in spite of no-smoking signs on the tables or have allowed cigars to be smoked, or have offered ash trays to individuals sitting at tables with no-smoking signs.

✔ . . .We are told that smoking policy enforcement is up to the individual ship's captain and so is not in control of the company.

✔ . . .And we are told that the company's policy controls the ship's policy, but that enforcement can vary.

✔ . . .And we are also told that the company's policy controls, period.

✔ Try asking for written confirmation of the smoking policy on board the ship you have selected and a refund in case the policy has been misrepresented. You may then be able to use the letter as leverage on board the ship if you need to.

The good news is that cruise lines are beginning to announce new no-smoking policies. As lines that carry mostly American passengers listen to those passengers' requests, we may be seeing more stringent smoking policies.

> Designating cabins as non-smoking cabins means that a greater percentage of smokers will use the smoking cabins than would ordinarily be the case. The result of this is that smoke odor in smoking cabins is more intense. If you cannot book passage in a smoke-free cabin, you should consider carefully whether or not you want to take the cruise on that date.

American Hawaii, Carnival, Majesty, Princess, and World Explorer have smoke-free dining rooms.

The following is a list of organizations that offer information on environmental tobacco smoke. Some publish newsletters which keep you up to date on medical studies, state laws, and lawsuits.

Asthma Resources Directory

Environmental Smoke

ORGANIZATIONS

These organizations offer information on environmental tobacco smoke:

Action on Smoking and Health — ASH
2013 H. St., NW (APD)
Washington, DC 20006
202-659-4310
ASH Smoking and Health Review, newsletter

American Heart Association
7320 Greenville Ave. (APD)
Dallas, TX 75231-4502
214-373-6300
Fax 214-706-1341
Information on tobacco-related heart disease, stroke; smoking cessation programs

American Lung Association
1740 Broadway (APD)
New York, NY 10019-4374
212-315-8700
Fax 212-265-5642
Booklets, programs for smoking prevention, cessation

Americans for Nonsmokers' Rights
2530 San Pablo Ave. Ste. J (APD)
Berkeley, CA 94704
510-841-3032
ANR UPDATE, newsletter

Americans Nonsmokers' Rights Foundation
2530 San Pablo Ave. Ste. J (APD)
Berkeley, CA 94704
510-841-3032
Educational materials for adults, educational programs for schools

Group Against Smokers' Pollution — GASP
PO Box 632 (APD)
College Park, MD 20740
301-474-0967

National Cancer Institute
9000 Rockville Pike
Building 31, Room 10A24 (APD)
Bethesda, MD 20892
800-4-CANCER (422-6237)
301-496-5583

Asthma Resources Directory
Environmental Smoke

The National Heart, Lung, and Blood Institute
9000 Rockville Pike, Bldg. 31 (APD)
Bethesda, MD 20892
301-496-5166
Fax 402-0818

National Institute for Occupational Safety and Health
1600 Clifton Rd N.E. Bldg. 1 (APD)
Atlanta, GA 30333
404-639-3771

Smoking Policy Institute
914 E. Jefferson, #219 (APD)
PO Box 20271 (APD)
Seattle, WA 98102

Stop Teenage Addiction to Tobacco — STAT
121 Lyman St. Ste. 210 (APD)
Springfield, MA 01103
413-732-STAT (7828)
    Information on preventing teenage addiction to tobacco

National Cancer Institute
9000 Rockville Pike Bldg. 31 (APD)
Bethesda, MD 20892
800-4-CANCER (422-6237)

ORGANIZATIONS OUTSIDE THE UNITED STATES

Action on Smoking & Heallth
372 Cowbridge Rd. E.
Cardiff, S. Glam CF5 1HF
Wales

Action on Smoking & Health
109 Goucester Pl.
London W1H 3PH
England

Action on Smoking & Health
8 Frederick St.
Edinburgh EH2 2HB
England

Action on Smoking & Health
Ulster Cancer Foundation
40-42 Eglantine Ave.
Belfast, Antrim BT9 6DX
Northern Ireland

Asthma Resources Directory
Smoking Cessation Programs

SMOKING CESSATION PROGRAMS

PROGRAMS FOR ADULTS

"Breathe Free Plan to Stop Smoking"

Seventh Day Adventist Church
(Call your local Seventh Day Adventist
Church listed in the telephone book.
     Five-day plan to stop smoking

"Calling it Quits"
(Call your local AHA for availability)
Available from:
American Heart Assn. National Center
7320 Greenville Ave. (APD)
Dallas, TX 75231-4599
214-373-6300

"Children and Smoking"
(Call your local AHA for availability)
Available from:
American Heart Assn. National Center
7320 Greenville Ave. (APD)
Dallas, TX 75231-4599
214-373-6300

"Death in the West"
     Video shows real cowboys dying of
cigarette-related diseases; available in
English, Spanish, Portuguese, Russian
Available from:
Narcotics Health Connection Catalog,
12501 Old Columbia Pike (APD)
Silver Spring, MD 20904-6600
800-548-8700
301-680-6740

"Expectant Parent Activity Book"
Available from:
American Cancer Soc., Inc.
1599 Clifton Rd. NE (APD)
Atlanta, GA 30329-4251
404-320-3333

"Expectant Parent Facilitator's Handbook"
Available from:
American Cancer Soc., Inc.

1599 Clifton Rd. NE (APD)
Atlanta, GA 30329-4251
404-320-3333

"Expectant Parent Training Guide"
Available from:
American Cancer Soc., Inc.
1599 Clifton Rd. NE (APD)
Atlanta, GA 30329-4251
404-320-3333

"Freedom from Smoking®"
At Work Program - Team up for
Freedom from Smoking
     Multi-component smoking
education, cessation, policy
development program for the
workplace; includes implementation
package, company coordinator guide,
smoking cessation and maintenance
kit; Teammate Support Kit
Available from:
American Lung Assn.
800-LUNG-USA (5864-872)
Refers to local ALA for information

"Fresh Start Quit Smoking Program"
(Call your local ACS for availability)
     Three week class with facilitator,
participants, guide
Available from:
American Cancer Soc., Inc.
1599 Clifton Rd. NE (APD)
Atlanta, GA 30329-4251
404-320-3333

"Freshstart Participant's Guide"
Available from:
American Cancer Soc., Inc.
1599 Clifton Rd. NE (APD)
Atlanta, GA 30329-4251
404-320-3333

Asthma Resources Directory
Smoking Cessation Programs

"Healthy Beginning, A: The Smoke-free Family Guide for New Parents"

Focus on risk to infants, children from second-hand smoke; for new parents, health care professionals have a special edition
Available from:
American Lung Assn.
800-LUNG-USA (5864-872)
Refers to local ALA for information

"How to Beat Cigarettes"

Video illustrating methods and suggestions on how to stop smoking; relapse is discussed
Available from:
Narcotics Health Connection Catalog,
12501 Old Columbia Pike (APD)
Silver Spring, MD 20904-6600
800-548-8700
301-680-6740

"I Am Joe's Lung"

Video for grade 7 to adult uses animation and x-ray photography to show lung function and smoke damage
Available from:
Narcotics Health Connection Catalog,
12501 Old Columbia Pike (APD)
Silver Spring, MD 20904-6600
800-548-8700
301-680-6740

"If You Smoke, Please Try Quitting"

Audio cassette, handbook to help you quit smoking
Available from:
Pulmonary Paper, The
PO Box 877 (APD)
Ormand Beach, FL 32175
800-950-3698
904-673-7501
Fax 904-673-5044

"In Control: Freedom from Smoking®"

Video for home, office, in conjunction with freedom from smoking manuals
Available from:
American Lung Assn.
800-LUNG-USA (5864-872)
Refers to local ALA for information

"On the Air"

(Call your local ACS for availability)
VHS tape explains how to achieve smoke-free work environment; considers costs, consequences, litigation, smokers' rights, implementation, enforcement
Available from:
American Cancer Soc., Inc.
1599 Clifton Rd. NE (APD)
Atlanta, GA 30329-4251
404-320-3333

"Public Slide-Tape Presentation"

Available from:
American Cancer Soc., Inc.
1599 Clifton Rd. NE (APD)
Atlanta, GA 30329-4251
404-320-3333

"Second Chance: 1 in 10"

Video tells story of pilot undergoing diagnosis and treatment of lung cancer through x-ray, biopsy, surgery; available in English, French, Russian, Spanish
Available from:
Narcotics Health Connection Catalog,
12501 Old Columbia Pike (APD)
Silver Spring, MD 20904-6600
800-548-8700
301-680-6740

"Secondhand Smoke"

(Call your local ACS for availability)
Humor and science prove tobacco smoke increases risk to nosmokers; components of side-stream smoke and mainstream smoke; effects on fetuses, babies, children; VHS

Asthma Resources Directory

Smoking Cessation Programs

Available from:
American Cancer Soc., Inc.
1599 Clifton Rd. NE (APD)
Atlanta, GA 30329-4251
404-320-3333
and:
Americans for Nonsmokers' Rights
2530 San Pablo Ave. #J (APD)
Berkeley, CA 94702
PO Box 668 (APD)
Berkeley, CA 94704
510-841-3032
and:
Narcotics Health Connection Catalog,
12501 Old Columbia Pike (APD)
Silver Spring, MD 20904-6600
800-548-8700
301-680-6740

"Secondhand Smoke"
Humorous video shows health hazards of sidestream smoke
Available from:
Narcotics Health Connection Catalog,
12501 Old Columbia Pike (APD)
Silver Spring, MD 20904-6600
800-548-8700
301-680-6740

"Smart Move!"
Available in 1/2" and 3/4" video
Available from:
American Cancer Soc., Inc.
1599 Clifton Rd. NE (APD)
Atlanta, GA 30329-4251
404-320-3333

"Smart Move!"
(Call your local ACS for availability)
VHS tape informs, motivates smokers to stop
Available from:
American Cancer Soc., Inc.
1599 Clifton Rd. NE (APD)
Atlanta, GA 30329-4251
404-320-3333

"Smoking and Pregnancy Kit for Health Care Providers"
(Call your local ALA for availability)

Slide and tape program with workbook discusses the effects of smoking on the fetus
Available from:
American Lung Assn.
800-LUNG-USA (5864-872)
Refers to local ALA for information

"Smoking: How to Stop"
(Call your local ACS for availability)
Video shows how one smoker stops; discusses, analyzes habit; substitutes for habit; helping others; what to expect after
Available from:
American Cancer Soc., Inc.
1599 Clifton Rd. NE (APD)
Atlanta, GA 30329-4251
404-320-3333

"Special Delivery"
1/2" video
Available from:
American Cancer Soc., Inc.
1599 Clifton Rd. NE (APD)
Atlanta, GA 30329-4251
404-320-3333

"We Can't Go On Like This"
Video vignettes for smoking intervention programs serve to spark discussion, role playing from NIH; leader guide; various formats; for sale or for rent from rental librarian
Available from
National Audiovisual Center
8700 Edgeworth Dr. (APD)
Capitol Heights, MD 20743-3701
301-763-1874
Fax 301-763-6025

"What You Need to Know to Stop Smoking"
Audio cassette information on health effects of smoking; techniques to stop
Available from:
Health Edco, Inc.
PO Box 21207 (APD)
Waco, TX 76702-1207

Asthma Resources Directory
Smoking Cessation Programs

817-776-6461
800-433-2677

"Where There's No Smoke"
Available in 1/2", 3/4" video and slide-tape presentation; different versions target employers, hotel managers, hospital and clinic administrators, and school administrators
Available from:
American Cancer Soc., Inc.
1599 Clifton Rd. NE (APD)
Atlanta, GA 30329-4251
404-320-3333

"Why Quit Quiz"
(Call your local ACS for availability)
VHS tape, 1/2" video, 3/4" video discusses immediate, long-term health benefits of quitting; audience: former smokers participate
Available from:
American Cancer Soc., Inc.
1599 Clifton Rd. NE (APD)
Atlanta, GA 30329-4251
404-320-3333

"Women and Smoking"
1/2" video
Available from:
American Cancer Soc., Inc.
1599 Clifton Rd. NE (APD)
Atlanta, GA 30329-4251
404-320-3333

PROGRAMS IN SPANISH FOR ADULTS

"Death in the West"
Video shows real cowboys dying of cigarette-related diseases; available in English, Spanish, Portuguese, Russian
Available from:
Narcotics Health Connection Catalog, The
12501 Old Columbia Pike (APD)
Silver Spring, MD 20904-6600
800-548-8700

301-680-6740

"I Am Joe's Lung"
Video for grade 7 to adult uses animation and x-ray photography to show lung function and smoke damage
Available from:
Narcotics Health Connection Catalog,
12501 Old Columbia Pike (APD)
Silver Spring, MD 20904-6600
800-548-8700
301-680-6740

"Second Chance: 1 in 10"
Video tells story of pilot undergoing diagnosis and treatment of lung cancer through x-ray, biopsy, surgery; available in English, French, Russian, Spanish
Available from:
Narcotics Health Connection Catalog,
12501 Old Columbia Pike (APD)
Silver Spring, MD 20904-6600
800-548-8700
301-680-6740

"Secondhand Smoke"
Humorous video shows health hazards of sidestream smoke
Available from:
Narcotics Health Connection Catalog,
12501 Old Columbia Pike (APD)
Silver Spring, MD 20904-6600
800-548-8700
301-680-6740

"Smoking and Pregnancy Kit for Health Care Providers"
(Call your local ALA for availability)
Slide and tape program with workbook discusses the effects of smoking on the fetus
Available from:
American Lung Assn.
800-LUNG-USA (5864-872)
Refers to local ALA for information

"Time to Stop is Now"
16mm film on smoking cessation
Available from:

Asthma Resources Directory

Smoking Cessation Programs

American Cancer Soc., Inc.
1599 Clifton Rd. NE (APD)
Atlanta, GA 30329-4251
404-320-3333

PROGRAMS FOR CHILDREN

"ACS Health Network"
(Call your local ACS for availability)
Teaching kit for grades 4-6; includes film strips, teaching plans, audio cassettes, activities for smoking prevention
Available from:
American Cancer Soc., Inc.
1599 Clifton Rd. NE (APD)
Atlanta, GA 30329-4251
404-320-3333

"Breathing Easy"
Film/videotape, teaching guide, books let teaches how respiratory system works; anti-smoking message; 5-8 grade
Available from:
American Lung Assn.
800-LUNG-USA (5864-872)
Refers to local ALA for information

"Breathing Easy"
Game show followed by talk show teaches the effects of smoking on the body and health dangers; video; 4-10 grade
Available from:
Narcotics Health Connection Catalog, The
12501 Old Columbia Pike (APD)
Silver Spring, MD 20904-6600
800-548-8700
301-680-6740

"Death in the West"
Film and curriculum guide
Available from:
Americans for Nonsmokers' Rights
2530 San Pablo Ave. #J (APD)
Berkeley, CA 94702
PO Box 668 (APD)
Berkeley, CA 94704
510-841-3032

"Death in the West"
Video shows real cowboys dying of cigarette-related diseases; available in English, Spanish, Portuguese, Russian
Available from:
Narcotics Health Connection Catalog,
12501 Old Columbia Pike (APD)
Silver Spring, MD 20904-6600
800-548-8700
301-680-6740

"Early Start to Good Health, An"
(Call your local ACS for availability)
Teaching kit for kindergarten through 3rd grade; includes teaching plans, film strips, audiocassettes, activities for smoking prevention
Available from:
American Cancer Soc., Inc.
1599 Clifton Rd. NE (APD)
Atlanta, GA 30329-4251
404-320-3333

"Health Myself"
(Call your local ACS for availability)
Three teaching units on smoking prevention, personal health; designed to be used in an integrated social studies, science, language arts program for grades 7-9
Available from:
American Cancer Soc., Inc.
1599 Clifton Rd. NE (APD)
Atlanta, GA 30329-4251
404-320-3333

"Healthy Decisions"
(Call your local ACS for availability)
Apple computer software program for grades 4-6; involves long-term effects of current decisions
Available from:
American Cancer Soc., Inc.
1599 Clifton Rd. NE (APD)
Atlanta, GA 30329-4251
404-320-3333

Asthma Resources Directory
Smoking Cessation Programs

"Huffless, Puffless Dragon"
(Call your local ACS for availability)

Animated cartoon emphasizes hazards of cigarette smoking; video; K-6
Available from:
American Cancer Soc., Inc.
1599 Clifton Rd. NE (APD)
Atlanta, GA 30329-4251
404-320-3333

"Hugh McCabe: The Coach's Final Lesson"
Smoking prevention program for middle school and junior high school students; teachers' guide, videotape/film
Available from:
American Lung Assn.
800-LUNG-USA (5864-872)
Refers to local ALA for information

"I Am Joe's Lung"
Video for grade 7 to adult uses animation and x-ray photography to show lung function and smoke damage
Available from:
Narcotics Health Connection Catalog, The
12501 Old Columbia Pike (APD)
Silver Spring, MD 20904-6600
800-548-8700
301-680-6740

"Lungs Are for Life"
Kit for teachers on smoking prevention; units on smoking, air pollution, lung physiology for K-4; activities, games, posters
Available from:
American Lung Assn.
800-LUNG-USA (5864-872)
Refers to local ALA for information

"Marijuana: A Second Look"
Teaching guide for high school students, parents; includes activities, newsletter; features cast of TV show, "FAME," 9 to 11 years
Available from:

American Lung Assn.
800-LUNG-USA (5864-872)
Refers to local ALA for information

"Octopuff in Kumquat"
Smoking prevention film and videotape for children ages 4-8; booklet
Available from:
American Lung Assn.
800-LUNG-USA (5864-872)
Refers to local ALA for information

"Rex Ronan: Experimental Surgeon"
Video game hero shrinks in size and enters the body of a long-term smoker to repair smoking damage; correct responses to questions give players the tools to save the patient's life; runs on Super Nintendo Entertainment System Available from Raya Systems
2570 W. El Camino Real #309 (APD)
Mountain View, CA 94040
800-276-HERO (4376)

"School Anti-Smoking Program"
Speakers visit classroom to discuss the dangers of smoking; geared to grades 4 to 8
Available from:
American Lung Assn.
800-LUNG-USA (5864-872)
Refers to local ALA for information

"School Health Education Program"
Effect of smoking on lungs; coloring books, puzzles, mannequin, lung specimens; films; video cassettes; versions appropriate to each grade level
Available from:
American Lung Assn.
800-LUNG-USA (5864-872)
Refers to local ALA for information

"Second Chance: 1 in 10"
Video tells story of pilot undergoing diagnosis and treatment of

Asthma Resources Directory
Smoking Cessation Programs

lung cancer through x-ray, biopsy, surgery; available in English, French, Russian, Spanish
Available from:
Narcotics Health Connection Catalog, 12501 Old Columbia Pike (APD)
Silver Spring, MD 20904-6600
800-548-8700
301-680-6740

"Secondhand Smoke"
Humorous video shows health hazards of sidestream smoke
Available from:
Narcotics Health Connection Catalog, 12501 Old Columbia Pike (APD)
Silver Spring, MD 20904-6600
800-548-8700
301-680-6740

"Smoke-free Class of 2000"
Educational kit with anti-smoking activities
Available from:
American Lung Assn.
800-LUNG-USA (5864-872)
Refers to local ALA for information

"Smoking-It's Your Choice"
Presents facts about smoking, secondhand smoke, addiction, respiratory system; disease; damage to fetus; video for grades 3-9
Available from:
Narcotics Health Connection Catalog, 12501 Old Columbia Pike (APD)
Silver Spring, MD 20904-6600
800-548-8700
301-680-6740

"Smoking: Following the Crowd"
Video for grades 6 to 8 uses computer graphics to show dangers of tobacco, including actual damage to body
Available from:
Narcotics Health Connection Catalog, 12501 Old Columbia Pike (APD)
Silver Spring, MD 20904-6600
800-548-8700

301-680-6740

"Super RT"
"Super Respiratory Therapist" and Smokebusters Club tell children why smoking is not good for their health; scripts, bags, stickers, T shirts
Available from:
American Assn. for Respiratory Care
11030 Ables Ln. (APD)
Dallas, TX 75229-4593
214-243-2272
Fax 214-484-2720

"You've Come a Long Way, Rene"
Portrays handling of peer pressure and advertising through story of Rene who wants to be a runner and doesn't smoke; video; 5-8 grade
Available from:
Narcotics Health Connection Catalog, The
12501 Old Columbia Pike (APD)
Silver Spring, MD 20904-6600
800-548-8700
301-680-6740

PROGRAMS FOR TEENS
"Biofeedback Smoking Education"
Comparison of pulse, tremor, skin temperatures between smokers, non-smokers in classroom; project for grades 7-12 demonstrating negative effects of cigarette smoke
Available from:
American Lung Assn.
800-LUNG-USA (5864-872)
Refers to local ALA for information

"Breath of Air, A"
(Call your local ACS for availability)
Video for teenagers discusses problems associated with smoking; grades 7-12
Available from:
American Cancer Soc., Inc.
1599 Clifton Rd. NE (APD)

Asthma Resources Directory
Smoking Cessation Programs

Atlanta, GA 30329-4251
404-320-3333

"Breathing Easy"
Game show followed by talk show teaches the effects of smoking on the body and health dangers; video; 4-10 grade
Available from:
Narcotics Health Connection Catalog, The
12501 Old Columbia Pike (APD)
Silver Spring, MD 20904-6600
800-548-8700
301-680-6740

"Death in the West"
Video shows real cowboys dying of cigarette-related diseases; available in English, Spanish, Portuguese, Russian
Available from:
Narcotics Health Connection Catalog, The
12501 Old Columbia Pike (APD)
Silver Spring, MD 20904-6600
800-548-8700
301-680-6740

"Health Myself"
(Call your local ACS for availability)
Three teaching units on smoking prevention, personal health; designed to be used in an integrated social studies, science, language arts program for grades 7-9
Available from:
American Cancer Soc., Inc.
1599 Clifton Rd. NE (APD)
Atlanta, GA 30329-4251
404-320-3333

"Hugh McCabe: The Coach's Final Lesson"
Smoking prevention program for middle school and junior high school students; teachers' guide, videotape/film
Available from:
American Lung Assn.
800-LUNG-USA (5864-872)

Refers to local ALA for information

"I Am Joe's Lung"
Video for grade 7 to adult uses animation and x-ray photography to show lung function and smoke damage
Available from:
Narcotics Health Connection Catalog,
12501 Old Columbia Pike (APD)
Silver Spring, MD 20904-6600
800-548-8700
301-680-6740

"Let's Talk About Smoking"
(Call your local AHA for availability)
Film for secondary school children discusses effects of smoking on health
Available from:
American Heart Assn. National Center
7320 Greenville Ave. (APD)
Dallas, TX 75231-4599
214-373-6300

"Save a Sweet Heart"
(Call your local AHA for availability)
Interactive teaching activity leading to signed pledges not to smoke or not to smoke for a specified period of time; for middle school students
Available from:
American Heart Assn. National Center
7320 Greenville Ave. (APD)
Dallas, TX 75231-4599
214-373-6300

"School Health Education Program"
Effect of smoking on lungs; coloring books, puzzles, mannequin, lung specimens; films; video cassettes; versions appropriate to each grade level
Available from:
American Lung Assn.
800-LUNG-USA (5864-872)
Refers to local ALA for information

"Who's in Charge Here?"
(Call your local ACS for availability)

Asthma Resources Directory

Smoking Cessation Programs

Emphasizes effects of smoking on the body's respiratory and nervous system functions; video; 8-12 grades; for availability, check with local ACS office
Available from:
American Cancer Soc., Inc.
1599 Clifton Rd. NE (APD)
Atlanta, GA 30329-4251
404-320-3333

PROGRAMS IN SPANISH FOR CHILDREN

"Death in the West"

Video shows real cowboys dying of cigarette-related diseases; available in English, Spanish, Portuguese, Russian
Available from:
Narcotics Health Connection Catalog, The
12501 Old Columbia Pike (APD)
Silver Spring, MD 20904-6600
800-548-8700
301-680-6740

"I Am Joe's Lung"

Video for grade 7 to adult uses animation and x-ray photography to show lung function and smoke damage
Available from:
Narcotics Health Connection Catalog, The
12501 Old Columbia Pike (APD)
Silver Spring, MD 20904-6600
800-548-8700
301-680-6740

"Rex Ronan: Experimental Surgeon"

Video game hero shrinks in size and enters the body of a long-term smoker to repair smoking damage; correct responses to questions give players the tools to save the patient's life; runs on Super Nintendo Entertainment System Available from Raya Systems
2570 W. El Camino Real #309 (APD)

Mountain View, CA 94040
800-276-HERO (4376)

"Second Chance: 1 in 10"

Video tells story of pilot undergoing diagnosis and treatment of lung cancer through x-ray, biopsy, surgery; available in English, French, Russian, Spanish
Available from:
Narcotics Health Connection Catalog, The
12501 Old Columbia Pike (APD)
Silver Spring, MD 20904-6600
800-548-8700
301-680-6740

"Secondhand Smoke"

Humorous video shows health hazards of sidestream smoke
Available from:
Narcotics Health Connection Catalog, The
12501 Old Columbia Pike (APD)
Silver Spring, MD 20904-6600
800-548-8700
301-680-6740

READING MATERIALS

"Smokefree Workplace, A"
Available from:
Americans for Nonsmokers' Rights
2530 San Pablo Ave. #J (APD)
Berkeley, CA 94702
PO Box 668 (APD)
Berkeley, CA 94704
510-841-3032

"Airline Complaint Kit"
Available from:
Action on Smoking and Health
2013 H St. N.W. (APD)
Washington, DC 20006
202-659-4310

"ASH Legal Notice to Business"
Available from:
Action on Smoking and Health

Asthma Resources Directory
Smoking Cessation Programs

2013 H St. N.W. (APD)
Washington, DC 20006
202-659-4310

"Catalogue of Nonsmoking Hotel Rooms"
Available from:
Down Home Computer Services
5713 Sam Houston Cir. (APD)
Austin, TX 78731

"Cessation and Quitting"
Available from:
Action on Smoking and Health
2013 H St. N.W. (APD)
Washington, DC 20006
202-659-4310

"Cigarette Smoking and Health"
Available from:
American Lung Assn.
800-LUNG-USA (5864-872)
Refers to local ALA for information

"Clearing the Air at Work"
Available from:
Americans for Nonsmokers' Rights
2530 San Pablo Ave. #J (APD)
Berkeley, CA 94702
PO Box 668 (APD)
Berkeley, CA 94704
510-841-3032

"Custody Cases"
(Involving smoking and nonsmoking parents)
Available from:
Action on Smoking and Health
2013 H St. N.W. (APD)
Washington, DC 20006
202-659-4310

"Effects of Passive Smoking"
Available from:
Action on Smoking and Health
2013 H St. N.W. (APD)
Washington, DC 20006
202-659-4310

"End the Smoking Affair"
Available from:
Krames Communications
1100 Grundy Ln. (APD)
San Bruno, CA 94066-3030
800-333-3032

"Escape the Smoking Habit"
Available from:
Krames Communications
1100 Grundy Ln. (APD)
San Bruno, CA 94066-3030
800-333-3032

"Facts About...How to Keep Your Lungs Healthy, The"
Available from:
American Lung Assn.
800-LUNG-USA (5864-872)
Refers to local ALA for information

"Facts About...Second-Hand Smoke, The"
Available from:
American Lung Assn.
800-LUNG-USA (5864-872)
Refers to local ALA for information

"Freedom from Smoking® for You and Your Baby"
Available from:
American Lung Assn.
800-LUNG-USA (5864-872)
Refers to local ALA for information

"Freedom from Smoking® for You and Your Family"
Available from:
American Lung Assn.
800-LUNG-USA (5864-872)
Refers to local ALA for information

"Freedom from Smoking® in 20 Days Quit Smoking Manual"
Available from:
American Lung Assn.
800-LUNG-USA (5864-872)
Refers to local ALA for information

233

Asthma Resources Directory

Smoking Cessation Programs

"Freshstart Facilitator's Guide"
Available from:
American Cancer Soc., Inc.
1599 Clifton Rd. NE (APD)
Atlanta, GA 30329-4251
404-320-3333

"Freshstart Participant's Progress Guide"
Available from:
American Cancer Soc., Inc.
1599 Clifton Rd. NE (APD)
Atlanta, GA 30329-4251
404-320-3333

"Health Effects of Smoking on Children"
Available from:
American Lung Assn.
800-LUNG-USA (5864-872)
Refers to local ALA for information

"Health Hazards to Smokers"
Available from:
Action on Smoking and Health
2013 H St. N.W. (APD)
Washington, DC 20006
202-659-4310

"Hooked, But Not Helpless"
Patricia Allison
Available from:
Pulmonary Paper, The
PO Box 877 (APD)
Ormand Beach, FL 32175
800-950-3698
904-673-7501
Fax 904-673-5044

"How to Quit Cigarettes"
Available from:
American Cancer Soc., Inc.
1599 Clifton Rd. NE (APD)
Atlanta, GA 30329-4251
404-320-3333

"How to Stop Smoking and Breathe Free"
　　Steps to stopping smoking
Available from:

Narcotics Health Connection Catalog,
12501 Old Columbia Pike (APD)
Silver Spring, MD 20904-6600
800-548-8700
301-680-6740

"If You Smoke Take this Risk Test"
Available from:
American Cancer Soc., Inc.
1599 Clifton Rd. NE (APD)
Atlanta, GA 30329-4251
404-320-3333

"International Organizations"
Available from:
Action on Smoking and Health
2013 H St. N.W. (APD)
Washington, DC 20006
202-659-4310

"Involuntary Smoking: Risks for Nonsmokers"
Public Affairs Pamphlet
Available from:
Group Against Smokers' Pollution
(GASP®)
PO Box 632 (APD)
College Park, MD 20741-0632
301-459-4791
Can leave message on machine

"Let's Take Action on Smoking & Health"
Available from:
Action on Smoking and Health
2013 H St. N.W. (APD)
Washington, DC 20006
202-659-4310

"Lifetime of Freedom from Smoking®, A"
Available from:
American Lung Assn.
800-LUNG-USA (5864-872)
Refers to local ALA for information

"No Smoking: Lungs at Work"
Available from:
American Lung Assn.

234

Asthma Resources Directory
Smoking Cessation Programs

800-LUNG-USA (5864-872)
Refers to local ALA for information

"Quit Cigarettes Live Longer"
Available from:
American Cancer Soc., Inc.
1599 Clifton Rd. NE (APD)
Atlanta, GA 30329-4251
404-320-3333

"Rights of the Nonsmoker, The"
Available from:
Group Against Smokers' Pollution
(GASP®)
PO Box 632 (APD)
College Park, MD 20741-0632
301-459-4791
Can leave message on machine

"Self-Help Reporter"
Quarterly
Available from:
National Self-Help Clearinghouse
25 W. 43rd St. Rm. 620 (APD)
New York, NY 10036
212-642-2944
NY City Referrals 212-586-5770
Fax 212-719-2488

"Smart Move!"
Available from:
American Cancer Soc., Inc.
1599 Clifton Rd. NE (APD)
Atlanta, GA 30329-4251
404-320-3333

"Smoke Around You, The"
Available from:
American Cancer Soc., Inc.
1599 Clifton Rd. NE (APD)
Atlanta, GA 30329-4251
404-320-3333

"Smoke-free Child Care: A Study Guide for Family Day Care Providers"
Available from:
National Maternal & Child Health
Clearinghouse
8201 Greensboro Dr. #600 (APD)

McLean, VA 22102
703-821-8955 Ext. 254, 265

"Smoke-free for Life"
Available from:
Krames Communications
1100 Grundy Ln. (APD)
San Bruno, CA 94066-3030
800-333-3032

"Smoke-Free Workplace, The"
William L. Weis
Bruce W. Miller
Available from:
Prometheus Books
700 E. Amherst St. (APD)
Buffalo, NY 14215

"Smokefree Travel Guide"
Julia Carol and Elaine O'Gara
Available from:
Americans for Nonsmokers' Rights
2530 San Pablo Ave. #J (APD)
Berkeley, CA 94702
PO Box 668 (APD)
Berkeley, CA 94704
510-841-3032

"Smoking in the Workplace"
Channing L. Bete Co., Inc.
Available from:
Group Against Smokers' Pollution
(GASP®)
PO Box 632 (APD)
College Park, MD 20741-0632
301-459-4791
Can leave message on machine

"Smoking Policy: Questions and Answers"
Fact sheets by National Cancer
Institute & Smoking Policy Institute
Available from:
Group Against Smokers' Pollution
(GASP®)
PO Box 632 (APD)
College Park, MD 20741-0632
301-459-4791
Can leave message on machine

Asthma Resources Directory

Smoking Cessation Programs

"Sources of Information"
Available from:
Action on Smoking and Health
2013 H St. N.W. (APD)
Washington, DC 20006
202-659-4310

"Special Report: Involuntary Smoking"
Available from:
Action on Smoking and Health
2013 H St. N.W. (APD)
Washington, DC 20006
202-659-4310

"Tobacco Smoke and the Nonsmoker"
Available from:
Americans for Nonsmokers' Rights
2530 San Pablo Ave. #J (APD)
Berkeley, CA 94702
PO Box 668 (APD)
Berkeley, CA 94704
510-841-3032

"U.S. Nonsmokers' Rights Groups"
Available from:
Action on Smoking and Health
2013 H St. N.W. (APD)
Washington, DC 20006
202-659-4310

"Workplace Smoking: Costs"
Available from:
Action on Smoking and Health
2013 H St. N.W. (APD)
Washington, DC 20006
202-659-4310

"You Can Stop"
Jacquelyn Rogers, SmokEnders
Available from:
Asthma Outreach Library
37 Pillsbury Rd. (APD)
Sandown, NH 03873
603-329-5301
and:

National Institutes of Health
9000 Rockville Pike (APD)
Bethesda, MD 20892-0001
301-496-4000
Fax 301-496-2443

READING MATERIALS FOR ADULTS IN SPANISH

"Smoke-free Child Care: A Study Guide for Family Day Care Providers"
Available from:
National Maternal & Child Health Clearinghouse
8201 Greensboro Dr. #600 (APD)
McLean, VA 22102
703-821-8955 Ext. 254, 265

READING MATERIALS FOR CHILDREN

"Coqui Likes His Air Smoke-free"
Coloring book
Available from:
National Maternal & Child Health Clearinghouse
8201 Greensboro Dr. #600 (APD)
McLean, VA 22102
703-821-8955 Ext. 254, 265

"No Smoking Coloring Book"
Available from:
American Lung Assn.
800-LUNG-USA (5864-872)
Refers to local ALA for information

"Smoking Stinks!"
Sticker for children with picture of unhappy dragon
Available from:
American Assn. for Respiratory Care
11030 Ables Ln. (APD)
Dallas, TX 75229-4593
214-243-2272
Fax 214-484-2720

Allergy Products Directory
Copyrighted. Reproduction Prohibited by Law. 1259 El Camino #254, Menlo Park, CA 94025

Asthma Resources Directory

Index

INDEX

237

Asthma Resources Directory

Index

Allergy Products Directory

Copyrighted. Reproduction Prohibited by Law. 1259 El Camino #254,Menlo Park, CA 94025

Asthma Resources Directory

Index

Our thanks to the
non-profit organizations
and the companies in the pages following
for their interest in this project

Asthma Resources Directory

Asthma and Allergy Foundation of America (AAFA)

America's leading organization for people with asthma and allergies

- Provides up-to-date, practical and timely articles in our newsletter,
- Sponsors a nationwide network of local chapters,
- Offers peer support through 145 local, affiliated support groups,
- Funds important medical research,
- Maintains a large clearinghouse of current and affordable educational materials,
- Advocates on behalf of the 50 million Americans with asthma and allergies,
- Offers special services to physicians and allied health professionals.

Call or write:

Asthma and Allergy Foundation of America
1125 15th Street, NW Suite 502
Washington, DC 20005
(202) 466-7643 or (800) 7-ASTHMA
(202) 466-8940 FAX

The Allergy and Asthma Network•Mothers of Asthmatics, Inc. (AAN•MA), is a nonprofit health education organization dedicated to assisting 50 million people with allergies and asthma and their families. Individual and professional memberships include the following benefits:

- A subscription to AAN•MA's monthly newsletter, *The MA Report.*

- A **10 percent discount** on AAN•MA publications, videos, peak flow meters, nebulizer accessories.

- Membership to the **AAN Pharmacy Program** offering discounts on medications.

- Toll-free **hotline** staff support.

- **Marketplace** - offering discounts on allergy and asthma products.

- Special medical **updates and bulletins**.

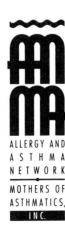

ALLERGY AND
ASTHMA
NETWORK
MOTHERS OF
ASTHMATICS,
INC.

Asthma Resources Directory

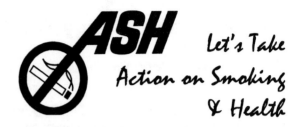

ASH *Let's Take Action on Smoking & Health*

99.98% of Americans smoke, whether they like it or not! We are forced to inhale other people's tobacco smoke—as a condition of holding a job, dining in a restaurant, shopping in a mall, or flying internationally.

Action on Smoking & Health is a national, nonprofit charitable organization that is supported entirely by tax-deductible contributions from individuals and private foundations. Using the tremendous power of the law to represent nonsmokers in courts and legislative bodies and before regulatory agencies, ASH has been successfully fighting for the rights of nonsmokers for over a quarter-century! ASH is responsible for cigarette commercial-free radio and television, smokefree flights and bus rides, and many other victories.

Yes! I want to support the work of ASH with a contribution of: ☐ $100 ☐ $50 ☐ $15✳ ☐ Other _____

☐ **SPECIAL OFFER:** we'll send the informative booklet "Taking Action to Protect You and Your Family From Passive Smoke" for an additional $3.50 (postpaid) — a 25% discount for Allergy Products Directory readers!

Name _____

Address _____

City, State, Zip _____

Your contribution to ASH is tax-deductible. Please make your check payable to ASH and send it to 2013 H St. NW, Washington, DC 20006 ✳ If you contribute a minimum of $15, we'll send you our bi-monthly newsletter.

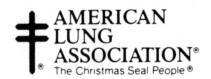

Asthma.
It doesn't have to restrict your life.

✝ **AMERICAN LUNG ASSOCIATION®**
The Christmas Seal People®

Asthma Resources Directory

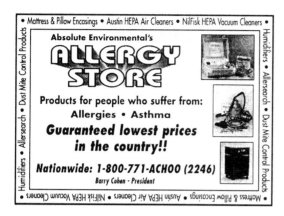
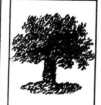

Allergy Products Directory
Copyrighted. Reproduction Prohibited by Law. 1259 El Camino #254, Menlo Park, CA 9405

Asthma Resources Directory

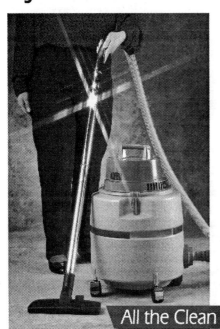
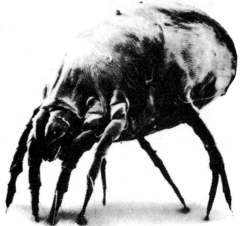

➤"Your Office Environment"

AAA Info Sheets help you recognize trouble areas, causes and symptoms.
Help you tackle the problems at work in a more knowledgeable manner.
Request Office Environment and enclose: $8

➤"Allergy Alerts from Living with Allergies"

American Allergy Association recognizes the special problems that you face in your daily life. *Allergy Alerts* gives you the facts you need to evaluate advertising that may mislead or misinform.

These alerts cover a wide range of areas from dyes in medications to medication interactions, food additives like sulfites, new foods like spelt, situations that could trigger asthma, problems with collagen, contact lens solutions, latex, even fabric softeners.

Be armed with the information you need to protect yourself and your family from misinformation or new products that may pose allergy problems.
When the news is too good to be true, you need the facts.
Request Allergy Alerts and enclose $11

➤"Pollen Times — By State, By Month"

Don't let your travel plans be ruined.
Don't compromise your business effectiveness.
Plan your business trip   Plan your vacation` Avoid pollen problems.
*Know **when** grasses, weeds, or trees are likely to be pollinating.
*Know **where** grasses, weeds, or trees are likely to be pollinating.
Request Pollen Times and enclose $7

➤"10 Steps toward Allergy Relief"

There are many things that you can do when you seek relief from allergies and these Information Sheets take you through the steps, helping you to make the decisions necessary for your medical health and well being.
Request 10 Steps and enclose $2 plus self-addressed, stamped envelope.

➤"Guide to Gluten-Free Diets"

Safe substitutes for baking and cooking
Differentiates celiac disease from wheat allergy
Sources of gluten in the diet. Warnings on when to check with the manufacturer
Buying guide for foods and ingredients — Plus a list of recipe books.
Request Gluten-free Diets and enclose $11

Allergy Publications
1259 El Camino #254 ●Menlo Park, CA 94025

American Allergy Association
Allergy Information Series — Practical Answers

➤ **"Eating Without. . .Packet"**

    12 Information Sheets describe the most common food allergens
    Specific problems with common foods and supplements
    The facts on milk ingredient labeling, milk allergy and milk sensitivity
    PLUS: 16-page handbook selected by Harvard Health Newsletter as a resource:
    Understanding Calcium and Osteoporosis
        Request Eating Without and enclose $11

➤ **"The New Labels"**

    Terms defined. What do all these new label words mean?
    How to more easily understand what the labels are telling you
    What are the meanings of the words that are used on the labels?
    Exceptions, Omissions, and Problems.
    What labels do not tell you. How the labels can mislead you
    Health Claims. What is allowed and what is not.
    Ingredient Labeling. Learn what must be listed and how.
        Request Labels and enclose $6 plus self-addressed, stamped envelope

➤ **"Infant Formulas for Allergic Infants and**
    Dietetic Concerns for Toddlers"

    How those differences affect testing, symptoms, and diet
    Misleading food labels — Reliable food labels
    What's in milk?
    When substitutes are suitable and when they are not
    Other formulas: Neocate, Whey or Casein or Protein Hydrolysates or meat-based formula
    Evaluating infant formulas
    Is protection possible for your child?
    What about elemental diets
    Other drinks: goat's milk, soy milk
    FDA labeling requirements under the new law
    Children under two — Children under four
        Request Toddlers and enclose $11

Allergy Publications
1259 El Camino #254 ●Menlo Park, CA 94025